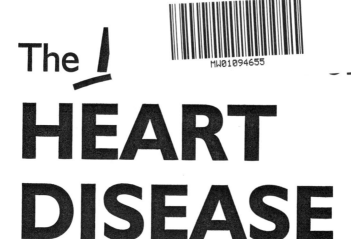

The **#1**

HEART
DISEASE

*Is **NOT** Cholesterol!*

"I lived the American dream. When I woke up, I realized I was living a nightmare. I had become a couch potato — the closest thing to a vegetable.

Smoking two packs of cigarettes daily, drinking and eating whatever I wanted, not exercising, all led me to be like the majority of Americans, obese and out-of-shape.

With a program, like the one outlined in this book, I was able to reverse the harmful effects of my own choices after I took responsibility for my own health. I discovered new vitality and overwhelming endurance. In the last 23 years I have run 700 races; 150 of those were 26.2 miles or more. I now live by the Greek ideal: Die young, as late in life as possible! You can too, simply by following this plan."

– **Roy Pirrung**,
World and National Ultra-marathon Champion, Member USA Track and Field Masters Hall of Fame, holder of 17 American Records

"When Paul Stitt asked me to do commercials for his new Natural Ovens bread on Chicago's WGN Radio in the mid seventies, we each had some stipulations: I wanted to know his complete story and he wanted me to try the bread.

Paul arrived at our studios one day with a big box of product and I interviewed him for two hours. The staff enjoyed Paul's generosity and I imagine the majority are still good customers even today. I know I am.

It was the interview that convinced me Paul was on to something and since our first meeting my faith in his research and dedication has not wavered. I am sure that not too many years from now, the medical community will come around and confirm Paul's theory that The Real Cause of Heart Disease Is NOT Cholesterol!"

– Roy Leonard,
Radio Broadcaster, WGN, Chicago

"If all the drugs were thrown into the sea, the fish would die, and human health would improve immeasurably."

– William Osler

The *Real* cause of

HEART

DISEASE

Is NOT Cholesterol!

by: Paul A. Stitt, M.S., C.N.S.

Contributing Authors:

Douglas Bibus, Ph.D.
The Holman Center for Lipid Research
Lipid Technologies, LLC
The University of Minnesota
Austin, MN 55912

Jeanie L. Burke, R.D. and L.D.
Swedish American Center for Complimentary Medicine
Rockford, Illinois 61108

Veronica Mocanu, M.D. and Ph.D.
University of Pharmacy and Medicine
Iasi, Romania

Natural Press
Manitowoc, Wisconsin

The Real Cause of Heart Disease Is NOT Cholesterol!

Published by Natural Press
P.O. Box 730
Manitowoc, Wisconsin
54221

Disclaimer: All information in this book is for informational
purposes only. None of the suggestions are intended to
diagnose, prevent, or treat a disease. It is suggested that anyone
wishing to make use of this information consult the relevant
resources and confer with a medical professional with expertise
in this area.

Substantial discounts on bulk quantities are available to corporations,
professional associations, and other organizations. For details contact
Natural Press at 800-558-3535 or visit our website at
www.realcauseofheartdisease.com

Library of Congress Cataloging-in-Publication Data

Stitt, Paul A., 1940-
The Real Cause of Heart Disease Is NOT Cholesterol!
Paul A. Stitt
p.   cm.
Includes bibliographical data on our website and index
ISBN 0-939956-10-1
1. Fatty acids in human nutrition. 2. Heart Disease 3. Medical
Institutions 4. Nutrition   5. Omega-3 fatty acids-Health aspects

Dedication

*To my wife, Barbara, who saved my life
with corrective nutrition
and who has been improving my health ever since.*

Acknowledgements

This work stands on the shoulders of some real giants in the field of nutritional biochemistry. The first giants were Drs. George and Mildred Burr who discovered in 1929 that Omega-3 (linolenic) fatty acids were essential. Then came Sir John Vane who received a Nobel Prize for his work on Omega-3 metabolism. I would also like to thank Dr. Hugh Sinclair, Dr. Artemis Simopoulos, Dr. Donald Rudin and Clara Felix (a team), Dr. Serge Renaud, Dr. Ralph Holman, Dr. William E. M. Lands, Dr. Andy Sinclair, Dr. Lillian Thompson, Dr. Bill O'Connor, and many others I have met at various conferences who have been very helpful at unraveling the many ways that Omega-3 work.

I would like to thank my colleagues at the International Society for the Study of Essential Fatty Acids and Lipids, American Oil Chemist Society, American College of Nutrition, and the Federation of Experimental Biologists for educating me in the arcane world of nutrition. I am deeply grateful for the many lively discussions at these meetings.

For helping put this book together, I am deeply grateful to Janet Brooke, Susan Akers, Sara Barnett, Charles Marwick, and especially Nancy Gratton for her help in editing this book.

Forward

Day after day I write prescriptions for cholesterol-lowering drugs. In a majority of cases I have pangs of conscience, knowing these chemicals will help my patients little, if at all. Worse yet, they may harm some.

My anger at being forced to do this started twenty years ago. A clever lawyer in California was able to convince jurors that the defendant doctor "had to be incompetent." He hadn't ordered a blood cholesterol test, even though the case had nothing to do with cholesterol. "Everyone knows how important cholesterol is!" the lawyer said, and he won.

Even then I knew cholesterol was a very small factor with respect to heart attacks. By addressing the major factors it would become even more insignificant. The highest incidence of heart attacks in the world is in a province in India, among people who have very low cholesterol levels.

Correcting the real factors for heart disease is addressed in this book. It would require, banish the thought, giving up some of our self-indulgent habits. Equally un-American would be the suggestion that it might require a little effort and discipline.

Unfortunately two things play a big role in medical care today. One is a false public perception of what constitutes good care, determined in large part by corporate advertising. In this case the real motive is not health, but profit.

The second determinant is the constant threat of litigation. All doctors feel threatened that if their patients' cholesterol is up even a few points, they must prescribe drugs or be held liable for any heart attacks. Again the determinant is not a health concern, but an economic one.

I met Paul Stitt in 1981 shortly after a return from two years of mission work in East Africa. Our teaching hospital served an area and population the size of Minnesota. The people did not have heart attacks. Clearly nutrition and life-style was a key. The insights and knowledge he has given me over the years have benefited my patients far more than the myriad of drugs I have prescribed.

Thank goodness for someone like Paul, who is willing to take on the drug consortium and help reverse the "quick fix" myth in our society that a pill will cure every ill.

William C. Dam, MD, SC
Internal Medicine
Westlake Clinic
Ingleside, IL 60041

Forward

My interest in coronary disease began in the 1960's. In 1968, I started my work in coronary artery bypass surgery. Pain relief in the patients was dramatic, even as soon as the day following surgery. For sick, poorly functioning hearts, immediate improvement in heart function was often dramatic following the new blood supply. It was clear from the start that bypass surgery improved the plumbing but did nothing for the basic cause of atherosclerosis. In those early years, American Heart cookbooks were given to patients and conventional low fat, low cholesterol diets recommended. There was never significant evidence that this diet did anything preventive for our patients.

An extensive database was established, and up-to-date survival data on over 98% of patients from 1968 to 1998 has been documented. In forty-year-old men with undamaged hearts, even with multiple arterial grafts, life expectancy after surgery does not begin to approach life expectancy of the general population of forty-year-olds.

Survival in sixty-year-old men after surgery just exceeds the survival of the general population. About half of the deaths in sixty year olds are due to coronary disease. If bypass surgery cured coronary problems, the post-op bypass patients should have shown dramatically better survival rates than the general sixty-year-old population. "Corrective" bypass surgery confers no unusual life expectancy but survival is clearly better than without surgery. Bypass surgery or angioplasty is important when needed.

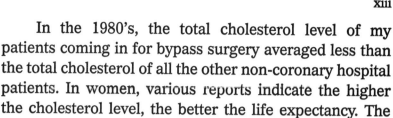

In the 1980's, the total cholesterol level of my patients coming in for bypass surgery averaged less than the total cholesterol of all the other non-coronary hospital patients. In women, various reports indicate the higher the cholesterol level, the better the life expectancy. The fractions of cholesterol, such as high or low-density cholesterol, do play a role in the incidence of heart disease.

Atherosclerosis follows multiple different events. When an excess of certain foods enter the body, oxidized or charged particles are produced. These particles damage the delicate lining of the arteries. In the natural healing process, the body responds by having platelets and white blood cells attach to the injured cells. Some white cells penetrate the arterial wall and stay there in the injured tissue. Then cholesterol gets deposited in the injured tissue. As the cholesterol piles up, the surface of the plaque breaks down. These raw areas once again cause platelets and fibrin to form and clot develops. The clot can rapidly develop, close off the artery, and a heart attack occurs. Cholesterol is a tiny aspect in this whole process. This book deals in ways to prevent the initial inflammation, prevent the progression, and reduce the chances of clot formation, which causes the final event. Most of this can be accomplished without expensive medications.

For your health, read on........

W. Dudley Johnson, MD
Johnson Heart Care Center
Milwaukee, Wisconsin 53005

Table of Contents

Chapter Two:
Science And The Medical Community _____29

Introduction

Given my background, it's probably not surprising that I have had a lifelong interest in quality food and nutrition. My father had a farm in Illinois where he raised grains, vegetables, cattle, pigs, chickens and other animals. All eight of his children, including me, helped out with the chores. We also grew up eating fresh, home-grown foods—with, of course, the occasional processed, snack, and convenience foods when they started coming onto the market back in the 1950s (treats bought for special occasions). Mostly we ate foods that we produced on our own land, by our own hands.

Farm-family values are strong values, passed down from parents to children. My grandfather had several adages, which he passed along to us. One of them was so much a part of his personal philosophy that it was inscribed on his tombstone: "He who helps others, lives not in vain." At an early age I had made this philosophy my own, and I knew that my life's work would involve helping others. After graduating high school I was determined to combine my grandfather's "helping others" philosophy with my interest in food production, because to me one of the most important issues of the day was the problem of world hunger. I decided that I wanted to become a scientist—specifically, a biochemist—because I felt this would be the best way to prepare myself to help solve this problem.

Because I was young, I initially thought the problem of world hunger had a simple cause: there wasn't enough food to go around. My early work taught me the problem was more complex and hunger isn't solely a matter of a lack of food, but a greater problem was (and still is) a lack of adequate nutrition in the available food.

After earning my undergraduate degree I went on to graduate school at the University of Wisconsin, where I undertook advanced professional training. With my newly minted Master's Degree in hand, I went out to find a job and wound up working for some of the biggest food producers in the country. It was there, however, I became aware my employers did not share my philosophy of helping others—in fact, I became convinced the primary objective of these companies is solely to make food that sells, and nutrition was the least of their concerns. Realizing this, I decided the time had come to part ways with corporate food producers and find a new way to put my experience, expertise and personal philosophy into action.

Along with my grandfather's philosophy, I had long ago taken to heart another bit of wisdom—one that came right off the cover of a workbook I used in grade school. On the cover of that workbook was a simple phrase: "Think and Do!" It's a simple idea, but a powerful one that has guided my life. I began to seriously think about how I could best fulfill my goals, and when I came up with a plan of action, I was ready to "do." The result? I began a new career: teaching people to understand nutrition and providing products that I knew to be natural, affordable, and health giving. To carry out this plan, I founded the Natural Ovens Bakeries of Manitowoc, Wisconsin, and Valparaiso, Indiana.

A Worsening Problem

My leaving the big, commercial food producers didn't bring an end to the corporate philosophy that focuses on "what sells." It still prevails in the marketplace today—if anything, it's gotten worse, not better, since the days when I said goodbye to my last "mainstream" job. You can see evidence of this attitude in every food ad that appears in magazines and on TV. The ads aren't about nutrition—they are about lifestyle and fun. By shifting the focus away from nutrition, the 'food' producers do not have to admit their foods are processed in ways that eliminate virtually all of the nutrition in them. They can sell foods which are loaded with things that are simply not good for you: preservatives, artificial sweeteners, flavoring and colorings, partially hydrogenated (trans) fats, refined white flour, high salt and sugar—because they put all their marketing into claiming their foods "taste good," instead of promising their foods are good for you. Do their processed foods taste good? You bet! In fact, the food tastes so good that you want more and more. Right?

Tasting good is only a part of why you choose foods. Your body needs much, much more. It needs fiber so that you feel satisfied after eating, yet the processed foods are woefully lacking in fiber. It needs nutrients! After all, that's the whole point of eating, isn't it? To nourish your body! Unfortunately, most of the commercially prepared, processed, and fast foods will never satisfy you and give you the real nutrition your body needs. Not only that, these refined, processed 'foods' can do your body great harm.

Spreading the Word

I have devoted my career to trying to educate consumers about nutrition, but late in the year 2000, I started to feel frustrated. It struck me that even though we have crossed over into a new millennium; our understandings of nutrition and real health remain way behind the times. We have rampant obesity in this country—some are even calling it an epidemic—and heart disease is the major cause of premature death. This last point is important to me, because my genealogical tree shows that most of my forefathers died of heart disease and I didn't want to wind up suffering the same fate. With insurance costs reaching out-of-sight levels, it just makes plain good sense to do everything I can to live without illness.

Learning the Truth

While learning everything I could about maximizing heart health, I came across a lot of scientific research that made me very worried. I realized the medical community, pharmaceutical companies, and most sources of popular "health news" focused on just one issue: cholesterol. You are told there are pills to take, which will reduce your cholesterol. At the same time the food industry has started pushing anti-cholesterol messages on its products: "Fat Free" and "Cholesterol Free" seem to be the most popular phrases to be found on just about any kinds of foods you can imagine.

If you're wondering why this is a problem, then their advertising campaign has already gotten to you. The scientific literature paints a very different picture than the one offered by the medical community, malpractice lawyers, pharmaceutical companies, and mainstream food industry—a powerful economic conspiracy group that I call the Medical-Industrial Complex, or MIC for short. These people all stand to make a profit out of pushing the simplistic, scientifically dubious idea that to avoid heart disease all you have to do is avoid cholesterol in your diet and lower your blood cholesterol level. The problem is, if you buy into this "cholesterol theory," you are still dangerously susceptible to heart disease: all you'll accomplish is to go to your Maker with a low cholesterol count!

What The Science Says

Over the last twenty years, numerous studies have been done that not only show the cholesterol theory to be invalid, but also provide the nutritional information we need to develop a heart-healthy, low-cost diet. The problem is that most of this information is made available only in specialist journals. Even when it's posted on health and science sites on the Internet, it's usually presented in scientific language that is difficult for nonscientists to understand. I decided this would be a great way to put my "help others" and "think and do" philosophies into action: I could extensively research the current scientific literature on heart disease and compile my findings, then go through all the data and ask myself this question, "How can this benefit the average person?"

I came up with answers that form the body of this book. In each of the chapters, I present the available scientific knowledge about nutrition and heart health in straightforward, easy-to-understand language. I back these presentations up by directing you to our website, which has abstracts of the specific scientific studies from where the information has been drawn. Upon completion of this process, I came up with what I call the Maximum Quality of Life Plan. For scientific abstracts cited, you may access our website at www.realcauseofheartdisease.com. We will continue to update the website as new information becomes available.

Why Now

My desire to produce this book took on a new sense of urgency with the events of 9/11. That day was a wake-up call for many of us. We were all reminded that life is short, and we shouldn't put off doing the things we know to be important. Personally, this means that I felt it even more important to share my newly acquired understandings about enhancing heart health and prolonging life to as wide an audience as possible.

September 11th had an additional impact on my thinking about these issues as well. I have come to recognize that the people who perpetuate the cholesterol theory have done it by playing on our fears and our weaknesses—much the same way terrorists behave. They take our natural fear of dying and our reluctance to make major changes in our lives and use them against us: they hype the rising statistics about heart disease, then promise us that we can make ourselves safe from it by taking a simple pill. This approach, great for MIC profits, is not so great for us: their cholesterol theory continues to result in needless suffering and premature death.

Their goal is healthy profits. My goal is for you to be healthy! I want to help you educate yourself so that you will have the motivation and the confidence to assume responsibility for your own health. In other words, I want to help you to "think and do." I propose a partnership: using my scientific training, I provide you with the information you need in language that you don't need to be a scientist to understand. Your role in the partnership is to consider the information provided in this book and put it into action. Together, we can come up with an approach to diet, nutrition and living that will benefit your heart health no matter what your current physical condition might be.

CHAPTER ONE

Heart Disease And The Cholesterol Terrorists

For many Americans, September 11, 2001, was the first time they felt the threat of terrorist activity personally, and it has caused us to define terrorism in a very limited way: as the actions of some shadowy band of sneaks who are willing to cause mass death to further a political agenda. That is not the only kind of terrorism, and the motive for causing terror isn't always political. In fact, Americans have been terrorized for almost half a century by the activities of a group that has—directly or indirectly—caused far more damage than Osama bin Ladin's Al Qaeda.

I call these people the Cholesterol Terrorists. They don't deal in bombs or guns, but in a much more dangerously subversive commodity: misleading, oversimplified, and even downright untrue claims about your most precious possession–your health. Their goal is to keep every hospital bed filled, keep every surgery theater operating all the time, and to push every pill the drug companies can produce. They are not out to make political points; they're just out to make money.

Who are these terrorists? Your physician may be one of them. As a doctor, he or she doesn't make any money if you're so healthy that you never need medical services. It stands to reason that doctors' interests are best served if you see them regularly. But the family doctor is just the smiling front man for a much larger group, a group that includes hospitals, insurance companies, sue-happy malpractice lawyers, pharmaceutical companies, and even the big food producers. Collectively, this is the Medical-Industrial Complex (MIC), whose primary goal is to terrify us all into filling their bank accounts just as fast as possible.

The MIC and the Cholesterol Theory

The prevalence of cardiovascular disease–diseases of the heart and arteries–has been very profitable for MIC, which has come up with something I call the "cholesterol theory" in order to maximize their gains. According to this theory, cholesterol in the blood is the villain, and in order to prevent heart disease all you have to do is reduce your cholesterol level. The MIC has had great success in spreading this theory–just check the medical and health shelves in your local bookstore and you'll find dozens of books warning the public about the hazards of cholesterol. These are only the tip of the iceberg. The National Heart, Lung, and Blood Institute (of the National Institutes of Health) and groups such as the American Heart Association all issue pamphlets, brochures and Internet advice from their websites, and their message is the same: cholesterol causes heart disease. The MIC is terrorized by the malpractice lawyers. Physicians are scared to death, so they test every patient for high cholesterol and put them on cholesterol-lowering drugs for fear they may get sued.

What makes the claim that cholesterol causes heart disease so attractive to the Medical-Industrial Complex is that it allows the MIC to tap into the public's desire for "quick fixes." With the cholesterol theory, all you have to focus on is one simple problem–your cholesterol level–and you can fool yourself into believing that you're reducing your risk of heart disease. More profitably, the theory justifies the mass production of highly profitable anti-cholesterol drugs. The public likes to think that all they have to do is take a pill and the problem is solved. No need to change your diet, no need to change your lifestyle. A pill a day keeps the heart attacks away!

The problem is, *the propaganda isn't true!* Oh sure, if you take the drugs, you'll probably see your cholesterol level go down, but that's not the point. The point is to *prevent heart attacks,* and to achieve that goal, lowering your cholesterol is simply not enough. Two of the nation's most influential health and nutrition authorities, the FDA (Food and Drug Administration) and the AHA (American Heart Association), even admit that the cholesterol theory is inadequate at best. They say you need to follow a "good diet" along with taking drugs. The problem is that they have never defined what a good diet is all about. They don't tell you the biggest news of all: with a good diet, you probably won't *need* the drugs at all!

A cardinal rule in science is that a marker that correlates with a disease is not necessarily the cause of the disease. One must have a physiological mechanism to explain the steps. The cholesterol pushers have failed miserably to do so; however, the latest science shows that there are very logical, physiological steps to show how oxidative stress and nutrient deficiencies can lead to heart disease. This book will explain the details.

How Did the Medical-Industry Complex Brainwash You

So how do the conspirators within the MIC achieve their goal of brainwashing you into believing the cholesterol theory of heart disease? Simple:

- They aggressively advertise their "miracle" pills with *implied* claims.

- They subsidize studies that focus on the effects of cholesterol, and disparage or ignore research that challenges their point of view.

- They enlist physicians into their scheme through offers of free samples and other marketing techniques, encouraging doctors to favor their products.

- They scare doctors into recommending anti-cholesterol drugs by implying that money hungry malpractice lawyers will sue them for millions of dollars. The cost of such suits and the cost of malpractice insurance are so prohibitive that some doctors are leaving the profession.

- They strongly discourage patients from questioning their treatment.

The result? People like you and me, who really want to improve our heart health, are fooled into believing that our only option is to keep taking the pills and tests. When a heart attack occurs anyway, which is inevitable if all we're doing is taking their pills, we may have the satisfaction of knowing that at least our cholesterol level is low. But that's cold comfort while we're lying in our hospital beds—and it's even less comfort for our families if that heart attack is fatal!

Let's Look at History

For an example of how the MIC pushes its agenda, look at what happened in the early 1990s. Back then, nutritionists began a campaign to promote the consumption of oat bran, pointing out its natural cholesterol-lowering properties. Lots of people began eating oat bran, and the MIC noticed a sudden downturn in their sales of cholesterol-lowering drugs. After all, who needs drugs if you can get the cholesterol-reducing benefit from your food? The MIC quickly contacted a prestigious university and sponsored a study of oat bran's cholesterol busting abilities by comparing it to wheat bran, for which no anti-cholesterol properties had been claimed. Then they rigged the study. They ran the study using too few subjects, over too short a period of time, and gave their subjects an unreasonably small dose of oat bran.

Not surprisingly, the study gave the MIC the results it wanted: the portions of oat bran used in the research didn't seem to make much of a difference in lowering cholesterol levels in the blood. The MIC was quick to publish its findings, and to blare the news from every journal, newspaper, and television in America: "Oat Bran Doesn't Work!" The average consumer didn't know that their study was flawed, or that 32 other, unbiased studies had come up with the opposite findings. Overnight, sales of oat bran plummeted, and the MIC watched the sales of their anti-cholesterol drugs start to climb once again.

A Health Crisis in the Making

As mentioned earlier, the biggest problem with the cholesterol theory is that it misses the point. Using pseudo-science and highly selective, scientifically questionable evidence, it singles out the cholesterol and fat in our diets as the cause of elevated blood cholesterol levels, and then goes on to say that elevated blood cholesterol leads directly to heart attacks. The logic seems clear: take drugs to cut your cholesterol level (and buy foods marked "no fat" and "no cholesterol"), and your heart health is assured. There's just one little hitch: cardiovascular disease is still the leading cause of death in the United States, even at a time when Americans are paying the MIC $120,000,000,000 annually.

How big a killer is cardiovascular disease? It kills nearly *2600 people every day*—every thirty-three seconds a person dies of heart disease. This is virtually the same number of people (2823) killed in the September 11 terrorist attack on the World Trade Centers. Obviously, all that money we're spending on lowering our cholesterol isn't buying much in the way of heart health. Heart disease kills just as many people as it did 30 years ago; the only difference is that they are dying with a lower cholesterol level in their blood.

The tragedy is that these deaths from heart disease can be prevented. One estimate is that as much as 70 percent of heart disease can be prevented if treatment is based on the best available science, not simplistic, profit-motivated pseudo-research like the cholesterol theory. The fact is that if we ignore the MIC and its deceptive propaganda and take the time to educate ourselves about how diet and lifestyle affect our heart health, we really *can* reduce heart attacks, plaque, and the fatty deposits that line our arteries—and at the same time we *can* lower our medical care costs, ease the suffering, and dramatically reduce the number of deaths from heart disease.

Heart Health Statistics - How Bad Does It Have to Get

Cardiovascular disease affects us all. Consider these statistics from the *2002 Heart and Stroke Statistical Update* put out by the American Heart Association:

Deaths

- 61.8 million Americans have one or more types of cardiovascular disease; of these 29,700,000 are male and 32,100,000 are female. (That is 25% of our total population, including children.)

- In 1999, cardiovascular disease claimed 968,775 lives — 40.1% or one out of every 2.5 deaths in the US — and was mentioned on 1,391,000 death certificates (69%).

- In 2001, 512,904 women and 445,871 men died from one type or another of heart disease.

- Cardiovascular disease claims as many lives as the next six leading causes of death including all forms of cancer.

- About 150,000 who die from cardiovascular disease each year are younger than 65 years of age; and 33% of deaths from heart disease occurred before the age of 75.

- 35% of those who die from heart disease have a cholesterol level between 150 and 200.

Suffering

- In 1999, 6,344,000 patients were in a hospital because of heart disease.

- In 1999 there were 59,965,000 physicians' office visits related to cardiovascular disease.

Medical care costs

- In 1998 *Medicare alone* paid out $26.4 *billion* in hospital expenses for treating cardiovascular disease.

This data shows how big of a problem heart disease has become in recent years, but it only tells part of the story. For a more complete understanding of the problem, it helps to add a little historical perspective. Figure 1 shows how the incidence of death from heart disease has changed over the last hundred years.

The first thing you'll notice in Figure 1 is that since 1900, deaths from heart disease rose steadily for 60 years, and since 1965, they leveled off to between 700,000 and 765,000 per year–and these figures represent only deaths due to heart disease. They do not include deaths from high blood pressure or other forms of cardiovascular disease.

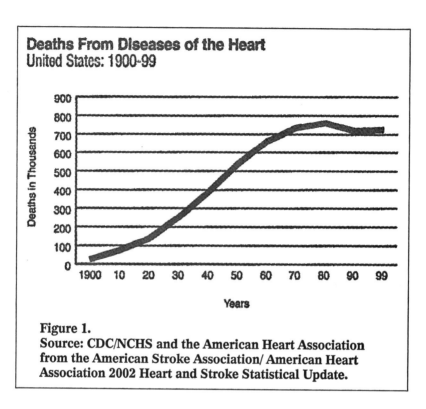

Figure 1.
Source: CDC/NCHS and the American Heart Association from the American Stroke Association/ American Heart Association 2002 Heart and Stroke Statistical Update.

Once Upon a Time,
There Was No Heart Disease

In the early 1900s heart disease was relatively rare, with about 10,000 deaths in 1905, the first year when such statistics were collected–compared to almost *1 million* deaths in 2001! Then between 1940 and 1960, something caused the death rate to start its steep climb and today it is an epidemic, in spite of massive expenditures on research and treatment in the last 35 years. How massive? Dr. James Anderson, of the University of Kentucky, reported in the June 19, 2000 issue of the *Journal of the American College of Nutrition* that Americans annually spend $120 billion for drugs, heart surgery including transplants and bypass operations, as well as related hospital costs, and this expenditure is rising much more rapidly than the annual average cost-of-living increase. But all this money has had a negligible effect on reducing deaths from heart disease. As a nation we are giving huge amounts of money to the MIC, but the American public is getting nothing back.

Let's return to Figure 1 and that steep rise in deaths that began in about 1940. What could possibly have caused such a dramatic change? It couldn't be genetic, because genetic change of this magnitude doesn't just occur overnight. We have to look elsewhere for the cause, at changes in our way of life that occurred during that era. When you think about it, the answer jumps out at you: this was the time when Americans made major changes in lifestyle and eating habits.

Eating More (and More Poorly) and Exercising Less

Early in the last century we ate three square meals a day and cooked at home. The food was natural in the sense that it was not refined, processed or loaded with additives. Today, however, the American diet is largely composed of processed foods that are heavily salted and loaded up with partially hydrogenated fats. Partially hydrogenated fats are a favorite of the food manufacturers because they give products a longer shelf life, and are found in most of the breads, cookies, and convenience foods that crowd your supermarket shelves.

The problem is that partially hydrogenated fats contain a substance known as trans fats, which have a tendency to form plaque in your arteries. In addition, every stage of processing that goes into producing convenience foods diminishes the nutritional content of the final product. When you add in the knowledge that around the middle of the century the great American love affair with labor saving devices and the automobile led to a dramatic decline in our level of physical exercise, a possible explanation for the increase in heart disease begins to make itself clear. A look at Figure 2 shows just how much our diets and lifestyle have changed.

Food	1900	Today
Grains	Whole grain bread and cereals only - white flour was not available for the masses	White bread loaded with preservatives, trans fats, and oxidizing agents
Meat	Unprocessed, fresh meat from animals raised on grass	Processed meat from animals fed Omega-6 rich corn
Vegetables	Fresh vegetables grown naturally	Canned vegetables or none at all
Dairy	Natural milk and cheeses	Processed dairy products with artificial coloring and sodium
Fats	Natural fats	Partially hydrogenated fats (trans fats) are in the majority of the foods on the grocery shelves
Salt	Salt available in natural foods and home-preserved foods	High salt snack foods are an every hour food item
Sweets (sugar)	Ice cream and desserts were eaten on special occasions only	High sugar, high fat foods are a daily staple
Drinks	Mostly well water	Mostly soda
Eggs	Free-range eggs rich in Omega-3	Factory eggs from hens fed mostly corn. Low in Omega-3
Exercise	Many types of work required physical labor	Individuals have 'desk' jobs and drive to fast-food restaurants

Figure 2.
Comparison of foods eaten in 1900 to foods eaten today.

Claiming that a change in lifestyle and diet has led to the rise in deaths due to heart disease doesn't really tell us what heart disease actually means. For that, we need to understand a little more about how heart disease happens.

Cardiovascular Disease: An Immune Problem

Recent research by Dr. William Castelli, director of the world famous Framingham Cardiovascular Institute in Framingham, Massachusetts, has shown that heart disease is really due to an out of control immune system. Reported in the November 26, 1998 issue of the *American Journal of Cardiology*, Castelli's research showed that malfunctions in the body's immune system can produce certain chemical compounds that cause lesions on the inner walls of the arteries. These lesions provide a place for soft plaque to attach itself. Calcium then infiltrates the plaque, causing it to harden—a process known as arteriosclerosis. Alternatively, a piece of soft plaque can break free of the arterial wall. When this happens the loose plaque is carried to another part of the artery where it can block the flow of blood. If the blocked vessels are those that provide blood to the heart, the result is a heart attack. If the blocked vessels provide blood to the brain, the result is a stroke.

The question is: Why does the immune system malfunction and cause lesions? And where does the plaque come from? There are many contributory factors, but research shows that the primary cause of immune system malfunction is improper nutrition: too much processed food and oxidized fat, and *too little of certain necessary nutrients* such as fiber, Omega-3 fatty acid (found in flax and fish), vitamins, antioxidants, and minerals. Too little of these nutrients can trigger devastating abnormal immune responses, then lesions, then plaque, then a heart attack or other cardiovascular disease. As for the plaque, we've already mentioned one source: trans fats, which are found in the partially hydrogenated fats used in producing many common processed and convenience foods.

Cardiovascular Disease Takes Many Forms

Now that we've explained what causes cardiovascular disease, it's important to recognize that it can occur in a wide variety of forms. Here are a few of the most common:

- Arrhythmia: Also called "irregular heartbeat," this occurs when your heart fails to maintain a regular, rhythmic beat, or beats too fast or too slow.

- Heart Attack: Death of heart tissue, caused by a severe lack of nutrients and oxygen.

- Angina: Damage to heart tissue caused by a mild deficiency of oxygen.

- Congestive Heart Failure: A weakening of the heart muscle due to nutrient deprivation or disease.

- Aneurysm: A weakening of the arterial wall that eventually bursts, much like a weak tire under pressure. Aneurysms can occur in any artery. Organs, such as the kidneys, can be damaged if their blood supply is stopped as a result of the aneurysm.

• Stroke: An aneurysm that occurs in an artery supplying blood to the brain.

• Arteriosclerosis: Your arteries are supposed to flex with each heartbeat. Arteriosclerosis is when they become stiff or hard (due to a build-up of calcium-hardened plaque) and can no longer flex with each heartbeat as they are supposed to do. Arteriosclerosis results in high blood pressure.

• Atherosclerosis: Your arteries become blocked, restricting the free flow of blood.

All of these problems can lead to death, sometimes instantaneously. Most of them are caused by nutrient deficiencies or a toxic overload of oxidized cholesterol, fat, or protein. So yes, there is a cholesterol connection to heart disease. But in most cases, cholesterol is but one of several contributing factors. Only a few types of heart disease are caused by high cholesterol alone. Nonetheless, the cholesterol terrorists continue to harp on that one substance as the major cause of heart disease. Why?

The answer is simple: there's money to be made, and lots of it. *As long as the public is kept uninformed about the facts of heart disease and the fallacy of the cholesterol theory, people will keep paying through the nose for high-priced prescription drugs rather than taking their health into their own hands and taking effective steps to reduce their risk of heart disease.*

Since you're reading this book, you obviously don't want to remain uninformed. You're ready to take charge of your health and do something constructive about preventing heart disease. To do this, it will help for you to understand cholesterol and the role it plays in your body, as well as how the facts about this substance have been distorted by the cholesterol terrorists.

Cholesterol: Lies, Death and Deceit

In the 1950's, Dr. Ancel Keys of the University of Minnesota advanced the theory that excess dietary fat and cholesterol were the principal cause of heart disease. Although there were those who questioned the theory, by and large the medical community and groups such as the American Heart Association seized on Dr. Keys's contention and continued to preach the theory for almost 50 years. It is the theory that still stands at the heart of the Medical-Industrial Complex's strategy for maximizing its profits.

The problem with Keys's theory is that it is an over-simplification of a very complex problem. Fortunately, there are signs that Dr. Keys's simplistic theory is being challenged in the mainstream press. For example, in the November 27, 2001 issue of *Time* magazine some fairly recent research findings about the causes of heart disease were reported as follows:

> As recently as five years ago physicians thought they had a pretty clear picture of what causes a heart attack. They saw it as a plumbing problem: too much fat in the diet builds up in the blood vessels that feed the heart, creating stop-

pages that starve the heart of oxygen. It was an elegant model and one that patients could understand. But it's not that simple. Cholesterol is just one part of a cascade of problems that can be stopped immediately by adding proper nutrients in the diet. Underlying the new research presented at the American Heart Association meeting was a clear message: This isn't your father's disease anymore.

But it's not just our understanding about the causes of heart disease that is changing. Its impact is changing too, for the worse. In fact, *it is striking people down earlier in life than ever before.* For instance, a well-known baseball player died of arteriosclerosis at the age of 33, shocking most Americans. But those of us who have kept aware of these trends weren't shocked at all.

The Rest of the Story About Cholesterol

The cholesterol terrorists have been so successful in their propaganda that most people don't know that their bodies actually *need* a certain amount of cholesterol. In fact, your brain cells, nerves, and many of your organs cannot function without it. It provides electrical insulation for your brain and nervous system, and keeps you from going crazy! Most people would be surprised to find out that even if they stopped eating all foods containing cholesterol, they'd still have it in their blood. That's because your body makes it, every second of every day, even if you do not eat any foods containing cholesterol. We would soon die if our body could not make cholesterol.

Cholesterol is often described as a fat. In fact it's a waterproof molecule, meaning that it does not dissolve in water. All mammals incorporate it into the walls of their cells, in effect waterproofing them. This is critical for the normal functioning of cells, especially nerve cells, which have the highest concentration of cholesterol.

Cholesterol Myths

In his book *The Cholesterol Myth*, Dr. Uffe Ravnskov, a scientist from Lund, Sweden, describes the role of cholesterol this way: "Cholesterol in the cell walls of living creatures leaves regulation of the internal cellular environment relatively undisturbed by chemical changes in the surrounding milieu." He goes on to say that cholesterol circulates in the blood inside particles called lipoproteins, which means that they are composed of a combination of fats (lipids) and protein. Ravnskov describes these lipoproteins as "submarines" that carry cholesterol through the blood.

There are several types of lipoproteins, categorized according to their density. The two most important types are the high density lipoproteins (HDLs) and the low density lipoproteins (LDLs), and they each are needed to perform specific tasks. LDLs carry cholesterol from the liver to the rest of the body, including the arterial walls, as it is needed. Ravnskov describes the process this way: "When cells need extra cholesterol, they call for the LDL submarines, which then deliver cholesterol into the interior of the cells." HDLs carry excess cholesterol from the rest of the body back to the liver, where it is stored for future use or–if it isn't needed–will ultimately be excreted.

Good? And *Bad?* Cholesterol

At any given moment, between 60 and 80 percent of the cholesterol in your blood is being transported by LDLs; another 15 to 20 percent is simultaneously being transported by HDLs to the liver. The rest of the cholesterol in your blood is being transported by other types of lipoproteins to other destinations. These days it seems that everybody has heard about HDLs and LDLs, and according to popular usage, the cholesterol carried by HDLs is called "good" cholesterol, while the cholesterol transported by LDLs is called "bad." But this distinction is misleading. Ravnskov explains how the "good" versus "bad" terminology got started.

> One may ask why a natural substance with important biological functions is called 'bad' when it is transported by the LDL from the liver to the peripheral cells but 'good' when it is transported in the other direction. The reason is that a number of studies have shown that a lower than normal level of HDL-cholesterol and a higher than normal level of LDL-cholesterol are associated with a greater risk of having a heart attack; and, conversely, that a higher than normal level of HDL cholesterol and a lower than normal level of LDL-cholesterol are associated with a smaller risk. Or, said in another way, a low HDL/LDL ratio is a risk factor for coronary heart disease.

Note that Ravnskov doesn't say that a low HDL/LDL ratio causes heart disease. That would be a distortion of the scientific evidence. There is an association between the two, but there are lots of other factors contributing to heart disease as well. It is just this distinction that the cholesterol terrorists ignore. They point to the association between HDLs, LDLs, and heart disease and *ignore everything else that might also be involved.*

The problem is, the cholesterol terrorists don't tell the public about all the other evidence that their "cholesterol theory" is leaving out. Most people, trusting in the pronouncements of authorities like the National Heart, Lung, and Blood Institute and members of the medical and pharmaceutical industries, have simply believed what they are told. That's why the majority of Americans have been willing to eat reduced cholesterol and low fat diets and to take drugs to control their cholesterol levels; believing that they are reducing their risk of heart disease.

If the cholesterol terrorists were telling the whole story, you would expect to see a steady decline in deaths from heart attacks. Unfortunately, this has not occurred. In fact, recent studies by epidemiologists have shown that eating low cholesterol foods or taking drugs to lower cholesterol does not greatly lower the risk of dying from heart disease, except for a very small minority of people (see Figure 3).

Cholesterol Theory Prediction Accuracy is One Out of Eight

Figure 3 shows the flaws in the cholesterol theory's claim that a high cholesterol level in the blood leads directly to dying from heart disease. Based on the data produced by the Framingham Heart Study, led by William Castelli, the figure graphically presents the relationship between total cholesterol levels and the occurrence of myocardial infarctions (heart attacks). The study was a well-designed, long-term research project involving thousands of study participants over a period of more than 40 years. It shows that the cholesterol theory of heart disease holds true in only 12 percent of the cases, where cholesterol levels are exceedingly high or exceptionally low. If your level is above 300, you are sure to develop heart disease. If it is below 150, your chances of heart disease are near zero.

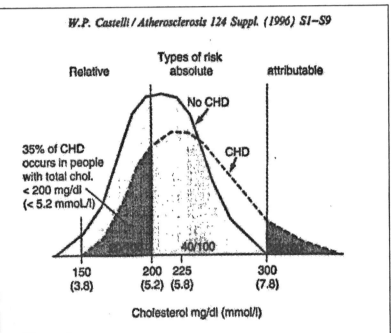

Figure 3.
The incidence of MI in relation to total cholesterol levels in the Framingham Study, 26-year follow up.

Castelli WP. Cholesterol and lipids in the risk of coronary artery disease — The Framingham Heart Study.
Can J Cardiol 1988;4:5A.

What does this mean? It means that for the vast majority of us, with cholesterol levels ranging from 150 to 300, the level of cholesterol in our blood is a very poor predictor of our likelihood of developing heart disease. The figure shows that 35 percent of all people who die of heart disease have a blood cholesterol level of less than 200, which many physicians cite as a safe level, whereas people who die with no heart disease have an average cholesterol level of 210. In other words, blood cholesterol levels seem to make no difference regarding the incidence of heart disease, except at the very extreme ends of the range of levels.

With this kind of evidence, which was first published in 1988, you might wonder how the cholesterol terrorists can continue to get away with their faulty science and their propaganda. There are several reasons why this has happened. First, of course, is the fact that we all want to find the "easy" way to solve our problems. If we can avoid changing our lifestyles by taking a pill or a potion, we're prone to do so. For people who buy into the low-fat, low-cholesterol diet mentality, there's another reason, too. They actually experience an improvement in their heart health, which convinces them that the whole anti-cholesterol propaganda machine is telling them the truth.

What they don't understand is that the improvements they're noticing is an accidental by-product of their anti-cholesterol diet. You see, foods that are naturally high in cholesterol and fat (animal products) also *happen to be low* in fiber, B vitamins, antioxidants, minerals, and Omega-3 fatty acids. Plant products are usually the opposite. Avoiding high-cholesterol animal products by replacing them with plant products greatly improves your intake of the spectrum of nutrients that really *do* protect you from developing heart disease. Unfortunately, if all you're thinking about is reducing your intake of cholesterol and fat, you might simply load up on "fat-free" or "cholesterol-free" foods instead of upping your consumption of plant foods. In that case you will certainly cut your cholesterol levels, but *you've done nothing to protect yourself from heart disease.*

A Better Way to Prevent Heart Disease

The point I've been making so far is that a low-cholesterol diet by itself does not and never will protect you from heart disease. It is only by raising your intake of a specific set of necessary nutrients that you can cut your risk of heart disease. This means that your best course of action is to quit worrying about cholesterol levels and concentrate instead on learning about the nutrients that really do make a difference for your heart health.

What are these *key nutrients?*

Here's the list:

- Fiber

- Omega-3 fatty acids

- B vitamins

- Antioxidants

- Minerals

Making sure that you get an adequate amount of these nutrients, plus making sure that you *drink plenty of plain pure water and get a reasonable amount of exercise* is your best strategy for reducing your risk of heart disease. Today's scientific research makes it clear that it is *increasing your consumption of these nutrients, not* reducing your cholesterol level, that really makes all the difference.

Back in the 1950s when the cholesterol theory was first proposed, it seemed so simple and believable. The problem is that even after 50 years and millions of dollars spent on research, no one has ever been able to prove it. That hasn't stopped the cholesterol terrorists of the MIC.

Don't be duped by the cholesterol terrorists. *There's no magic pill that will protect you from heart attack.* Using a drug to synthetically reduce your cholesterol level won't correct the underlying cause of the disease, which we now know to be a deficiency in key nutrients. Therefore, *you need to look at your entire diet,* not just the fat and cholesterol levels. In other words, you must determine why you might be at risk for heart attack and then correct the cause. Once you've done this you can relax in the knowledge that you have taken a significant step to reducing your risk of heart disease.

The Failure of the Medical Community to Deliver Real Health

As Americans, we like to believe that we're "Number One" in everything we do, so it's no surprise that most people cling to the notion that our healthcare system is the best in the world. People who believe this are in for a rude awakening. In July 2000, Dr. Barbara Starfield of John Hopkins University reported in the July 26, 2000 issue of the *Journal of the American Medical Association* that on 16 health indicators–including low birth weight, neonatal and infant mortality, and life expectancy–the US ranks twelfth in terms of good health out of thirteen of the worlds' leading industrial nations. "We rank above Germany, but *lower* than Japan, Sweden, Canada, France, Australia, Spain, Finland, The Netherlands, the United Kingdom, Denmark and Belgium," she said.

We have more military and industrial power than all these countries combined; but we are at the bottom of the list when it comes to *prevention* in the field of healthcare. We are not even in the top ten for life expectancy no matter what the age group—one year olds, fifteen-year olds, or forty-year olds.   What is even worse, we working Americans lose more productive work years of our lives than any of the other thirteen countries. We are simply sick way too often for being the world's most powerful country, and we hope, the world's smartest.

"The reasons for Americans' relatively poor health are complex and not due to a single factor," says Starfield. She suggests that one reason may be the failure of the American medical care system to build a strong base of primary medical care. She notes that of the 7 countries that are at the top of the medical care ranks, 5 have strong primary *preventive* medical care structures.

Starfield's findings point out a strange contradiction in the American approach to health and sickness care. We actively desire good health and greater longevity, but we don't take personal responsibility to get it. Instead, we rely on "the experts" to tell us what to do. Sometimes that turns out to be a good thing: we've done better than the citizens of most other countries at cutting out smoking and cutting down on our consumption of alcohol. Sometimes our reliance on "the experts" works against us, as when we accept without question the cholesterol propaganda put out by the MIC. That is because we forget that *our medical care system really does not prioritize health.*

The American medical care system has been described as a "sick-care" system, one in which the focus is on *treating* disease *rather than preventing it.* This is obviously the reverse of your priority and mine, which is to avoid getting sick in the first place. Unfortunately, even in terms of its own priorities, the U.S. medical industry isn't doing a very good job. In November 1999, the Institute of Medicine (IOM) issued a report on physician- and medication-related errors, which estimated that 44,000-98,000 Americans die each year as a result of medical mistakes. This number is thirty times the number of people that died in the World Trade Centers. The IOM arrived at its estimate by extrapolating from adverse events that occurred in hospitals in Colorado, Utah, and New York.

Hospitals Are Risky Places

In her report on the poor health statistics for the U.S., Starfield also noted the high rate of errors and adverse events that occur in everyday medical and hospital practice. She cited published reports that estimated there are 12,000 deaths a year from unnecessary surgery; 7,000 deaths a year from medication errors in hospitals; 20,000 deaths from other mistakes in hospitals; 80,000 deaths a year from infections acquired by patients while in hospital; and 106,00 deaths a year from *adverse effects of medications* but not due to mistakes. These total 225,000 deaths a year, a hundred times as many as died in the World Trade Centers. These mistakes are the *third leading cause of death* in the US after heart disease and cancer, and is due to patients either getting the wrong drugs or being treated for a disease they didn't have.

This is only part of the story. Starfield notes these figures cover only deaths; they do *not* include adverse events associated with disability or discomfort, or the pain and suffering people experience from drugs or treatments that were not serious enough to cause death. She cites the following startling figures: (annually)

- 116 million extra physicians' office visits

- 77 million extra prescriptions

- 17 million visits to the emergency room

- 8 million admissions to hospital

- 3 million long-term care admissions

The total bill for these extra costs comes to an astonishing $77 billion, and it comes out of *your* pocket in the form of higher taxes and medical insurance premiums. This is the *financial insult* that's added to the personal injury and pain you suffer from inadequate, faulty, or unnecessary medical procedures. The problem is, most of us are completely unaware of these failures in our health-care system. Reports like Starfield's are published in medical journals, but rarely are made available to the general public. While our governmental officials have access to this information, they have yet to act upon it. The MIC is a powerful group of special interests, and our politicians aren't about to antagonize it.

Now you know the truth. Physicians are not infallible and neither are we. The medical and pharmaceutical communities are not in business for the fun of it. Like every other industry, they're out to make a profit. This means that you can't count on them to always keep your best interests at heart. *You must take responsibility* and become your own health advocate. You must educate yourself about the best way to enhance your health.

In the chapters that follow, you will be provided with information that will enable you to do this. My own extensive research has led me to the conclusion that the single most important thing any of us can do to improve our health and reduce our risk of heart disease is to adopt the principles of proper nutrition. Unfortunately, nutrition is one area in which our physicians are not well trained. In fact, *traditional medical training overlooks* this very important aspect of *preventive health care*, focusing instead on disease diagnosis, remedial care once disease or disability has already occurred, and surgical or drug interventions. Only recently has the medical community begun to look beyond this traditional model and to include alternative medicine and nutrition in their curricula.

Until this nutritional trend becomes an established part of the medical establishment, however, we will have to take preventive action ourselves. When it comes to heart disease (and many other common ailments, for that matter) a big part of our solution can come from adopting a sound, informed approach to nutrition and exercise. By reading this book, you're taking that all-important first step toward that goal. Remember, no matter what your age, no matter what the current state of your health, *you have the power to vastly improve the quality of your life.* All it takes is a willingness to learn, and then to put what you've learned into practice: Think and Do!

– CHAPTER TWO –

Science And The
Medical Community

It has always been human nature to reject new ideas. New ideas represent change, and change is often viewed with apprehension. There always appears to be more security in the familiar than in the unknown. Physicians are no different than anyone else. That's why, historically, the medical community has been slow to adopt new paradigms. There's another reason for this conservativeness on the part of the medical community. Change can cut into profits. Physicians, especially those treating patients under managed care programs and under some health insurance plans, are often discouraged from trying alternatives to the established routine, which generally involve medications. Explaining alternatives to patients takes too much time. It's quicker and easier, and much more profitable, to write a prescription for a drug.

So it's no surprise that, in the world of medicine, progress often evolves with glacier-like slowness. Ironically, some of the greatest health breakthroughs in history were initially ridiculed, scorned and rejected for many years, then finally accepted by medical science as if they had discovered it. There are an ample number of examples from the history of medicine about physicians being slow adapters of new ideas and of *actually ignoring solid truths for centuries.*

Medical Progress Comes Slowly

The history of medicine is filled with stories of good ideas that are initially resisted by established authorities in the profession. One early example is that of William Harvey, who in 1623 discovered the function of the heart. Five years later he published *De motu cordis*, in which he described the heart as a mechanical pump that pushed arterial blood into the veins. The medical profession of the day totally rejected this finding, however. Many of Harvey's colleagues considered him a "quack" and criticized him savagely. At the time, physicians believed in the ancient theory that the only function of the heart was "to think and feel." *Today*, Harvey's findings are considered to be one of the greatest landmarks in medical research.

Vitamin C Rediscovered Three Times in 335 Years

Another example of the medical profession's reluctance to accept change occurred more than a quarter of a century earlier. In 1593, Sir Richard Hawkins, an English admiral, reported that the eating of either oranges or limes appeared to eliminate scurvy among his crew. He recommended that ships be provisioned with these fruits to prevent this disease, which killed thousands of sailors each year. "This is a wonderful secret of the power and wisdom of God," wrote Sir Richard Hawkins, "that hath hidden so great and unknown virtue in this fruit, to be a certain remedy for this infirmity."

The medical community rejected the Admiral's recommendation as being "too simple"! *It would take nearly 200 years,* until 1753, for Dr. James Lind to rediscover

Hawkins's advice. Lind started preaching to the medical profession how they could end this dreaded disease, but even he came under sharp attack and his views were totally rejected. It took over 90 years after Dr. Lind's death for the British Navy to make it mandatory for all seamen to eat a lime a day. In 1928, the medical profession was "forced" to accept Dr. Lind's theory just *335 years after it was first discovered!* In that year, the "anti-scurvy factor" was finally isolated. It is now called "vitamin C."

Cleanliness Before Godliness Took a Long Time Coming

Another case in point is the simple concept of anti-sepsis. In the middle of the nineteenth century, thousands of new mothers died of childbed fever. All of the greatest obstetricians in Europe believed the cause to be of "brought about by the local cosmic-telluric forces, the hygrometric forces, the polar currents, as well as radiation from the constellations. And finally: *the wrath of the spirit of the disease.*" However, in 1857 a Hungarian physician named Ignaz Semmelweiss discovered the real cause of childbed fever: the physicians were going straight from the autopsy room to the delivery room *without washing their hands!*

Dr. Semmelweiss proved conclusively that his theory was correct, and *lowered* the incidence of childbed fever in his hospital *by over 90 percent*. Yet the physicians still rejected his "foolish" ideas. He was even fired from his job! For the rest of his life he cried to all physicians "the murder must stop!" But very few listened. For almost nine decades after his death, tens of thousands of mothers died needlessly, all because the *physicians refused to listen to*

Semmelweiss and take the simple precaution of washing their hands!

Genetics Disputed for Hundreds of Years

The science of genetics is another example of how long it can take for science and medicine to work together. Around the middle of the nineteenth century, Gregor Mendel started crossbreeding several varieties of peas. He meticulously documented the characteristics of each succeeding generation. His simple findings represented the beginning of the modern field of genetics. Mendel's research represented one of the most important findings in science. At the time, his published views were totally rejected by his contemporaries, as no one was willing to listen to the views of an amateur vegetable gardener. It took almost thirty years before "real" scientists substantiated his work!

Vitamin B-12 Ignored for 25 Years After Discovery

The discovery of the cure for pernicious anemia was also ignored for twenty-five years. We now know that this disease results from a vitamin B12 deficiency that impairs the body's ability to make blood, accelerates blood cell destruction, and damages the nervous system. In the early decades of the 20th century, however, pernicious anemia killed more than 70,000 people needlessly, all because a doctor named George Whipple of the University of Rochester (New York) was ignored by the medical community.

Whipple was the first to demonstrate that foods, particularly organ meats like liver and kidney, played a role in the regeneration of red cells in the blood. In 1926, two Harvard Medical School professors, Drs. George Minot and R. William Murphy, based their research on some of Whipple's ideas and ultimately developed conclusive evidence that eating liver could cure this fatal disease; but they, too, were laughed at and ridiculed. As a result, the disease went on killing people.

For the next eight years, thousands upon thousands of people died of this condition. The physicians refused to give their pernicious anemia patients liver. In 1934, Whipple, Minot, and Murphy were belatedly awarded a Nobel Prize in medicine for their brilliant discovery, but even such recognition did not mean widespread acceptance. A year after the prize was awarded, over 8,000 people still died from the disease. It was only in 1950 that the death toll from pernicious anemia was ended. Twenty-five years after its first discovery, the medical profession finally acknowledged that vitamin B-12, the "anti-pernicious anemia x-factor" in liver, could cure the condition.

Bread Mold to Cure Diseases

Perhaps the most famous example of medicine's unwillingness to accept change occurred during the Middle Ages. Back then, millions of peasants all over Europe and China knew that a piece of moldy bread could cure an infection. Yet, for hundreds of years the medical profession rejected the concept that a "mold" could have such a beneficial effect. The medical physicians laughed at this silly idea!

In the 1880's, a French medical student named Ernest Duchesne discovered that a broth made from moldy bread could kill dangerous bacteria in mice. He presented his research to his medical professors. They read it and rejected it. What could have been one of the greatest health breakthroughs in the nineteenth century was quietly stuck in a file. It wouldn't be rediscovered for another 40 years.

In 1928, a Scotsman named Alexander Fleming "officially" discovered penicillin; however, no one in the upper echelons of science was much interested. One American university rejected an application for $100 to do research on penicillin. The university even threatened to discharge a professor who offered to pay for the investigation out of his own pocket! Orthodox medicine totally rejected the amazing discovery until the beginning of World War II, more than 11 years later, when the requirements of the military motivated the U.S. government to fund the project to make the drug widely available.

As a final example, consider how long it took for medical science to acknowledge basic information about human growth and development. Around the year 1730, a Frenchman named Henri-Louis Duhamel discovered how bones "grow" in the human body. Duhamel claimed that bone was laid down by tissue directly surrounding it. The problem was that Duhamel was not a scientist or a medical professional; he was merely a squire. Without official credentials, his "ignorant views" were bitterly attacked. It took more than two hundred years for the medical profession to be convinced that Duhamel was indeed correct! The tissue that Duhamel discovered is now called the "periosteum" – which is Greek for "around the bone."

Nutritional Training for Physicians: Less Than Sufficient

Like the insights and discoveries of Semmelweiss, Fleming, Duhamel, Whipple, and many others, *the latest research in nutrition is also being rejected* by the medical community. The subject isn't taught in most medical school programs, which means that your family physician probably knows less about it than the local veterinarian.

Consider this: in 1986, a study in the *American Journal of Clinical Nutrition* reported that three fourths of America's medical students were dissatisfied with the quantity and quality of their education in nutrition. In 1988, researchers reported in the *Journal of the American College of Nutrition* that nutrition scores in Southeastern medical schools for freshman were only 53 percent right and only increased to 69 percent for seniors. By the year 2000, a UCLA study reported in the *Journal of Cancer Education* found that test scores increased from 39 percent to 62 percent during the time from entering medical school to the end of the second year of medical school. There was improvement, to be sure, but the "improved" score was still so low as to alarm many educators.

This situation needs to change, and some medical programs are making the effort. The University of North Carolina developed a CD-ROM based program for teaching nutrition in 1998, and by the year 2000, seventy-six schools said they were implementing the program. Meanwhile, the University of Pennsylvania has inaugurated a nutrition program that is well-liked by the medical students and even has a textbook called *Medical Nutrition and Disease.*

In 1997 the National Heart, Lung, and Blood Institute developed the Nutrition Academic Award (NAA) Program, an initiative to improve nutrition training across a network of US medical schools. The purpose of this funding, which began in 1998, is to support the development and enhancement of nutrition curricula for medical students, residents, and practicing physicians to learn principles and practice skills in nutrition. The NAA Program constitutes a major new effort to enhance nutrition knowledge and skills among medical care providers and to effectively apply the science of human nutrition to clinical medicine.

Money and Prestige

Remember that it's not just conservatism in the medical community that inhibits change. There is also the financial incentive to stick to old ways and reject new ones. Modern nutrition science is not able to provide the profits that sticking with the old cholesterol theory can provide.

The cholesterol theory is a money-maker for the medical community for a number of reasons. First of all, it only costs a lab a few dollars to do a cholesterol test–but you can bet that it costs you (or your insurance company) a whole lot more. Yet the lab results are not very meaningful. Many things affect your cholesterol, so the value bounces around every day. You are encouraged to worry about it, then you're told to have it checked often–which just makes you worry more. With every test the medical community makes more profits!

The drugs used for *treating* high cholesterol are also

very profitable, and not just for the drug companies. Physicians do not get bribed to prescribe cholesterol-lowering drugs; however, they often do get lots of special considerations from the big pharmaceutical companies. Many drug companies will sponsor "educational seminars" on their products, held in some of the most faraway, beautiful spots in the world, and they foot the bill for the doctors who attend them.

There is a third reason that the medical profession is slow to make certain kinds of changes. Remember the story of Dr. Semmelweiss? One of the biggest reasons that his fellow doctors rejected his idea about washing their hands is that they felt it was professionally insulting. Something like that is true in the medical community today, especially when it comes to the link between nutrition and disease. For decades now, modern doctors have adopted the attitude that they are more important than anyone else who works in the health care profession. To be able to prescribe drugs or perform surgery is more prestigious than to offer advice on diet and exercise, which, after all, is something that "mere" dietitians and nutritionists do!

Lawyers Love to Sue Doctors

The simple fact is that your health should be more important than the medical profession's prestige and your doctor's malpractice insurance. You should have control over your health. If you are surviving on lots of drugs, then you are neither the master of your own health nor of your own pocketbook. You are at the mercy of the drug companies whenever they want to raise their prices. Before you can even get your prescription for the drug, you must have that high-priced office visit with your physician and he does a lot of laboratory tests to make sure greedy malpractice lawyers won't sue him. Doctors certainly should be protected from so many frivolous lawsuits for mega-millions of dollars. We're all paying a high price for forcing the doctor to practice defensive medicine. *How much better would it be if there were things you could do for yourself that would improve your heart health and do away with the need for these expensive physicians' visits, medically unnecessary laboratory tests and high-priced prescription drugs?*

There are, but before you can begin to do these things for yourself, you must move beyond the simplistic cholesterol theory so beloved by the MIC and really *get to know the facts about what really causes heart disease.*

Remember–the MIC has its own priorities, and your personal health isn't at the top of that list. If it were, we would not be one of the sickest nations in the world. Your physician would get paid only when he or she actually healed you and the drug companies would rush to make certain that their medications were priced as low as possible, so that everyone who needed them could afford them. You don't see that happening, right? You never see the MIC offering scientific proof that their anti-cholesterol drugs actually prevent deaths from heart disease. Even the information they do offer, like data on side effects, are provided in the smallest of small print. Physicians offer no guarantees–but too often we listen to them as if everything they tell us is absolutely true.

The Cholesterol Theory Revisited

Physicians don't offer the kind of proof and guarantees we just mentioned because there are none available. They can tell you, honestly, that high cholesterol levels are associated with heart disease, but that's all they can say. No research has ever shown that cholesterol actually *causes* heart disease all by itself. No research has shown the mechanism.

That hasn't stopped the MIC from trying to make you believe it does. For example, in 1984, the National Heart, Lung and Blood Institute of the National Institute of Health arranged a consensus conference with scientists who agreed that high blood cholesterol level is a major cause of coronary artery disease. The conference findings were summed up in these words:

> It has been established beyond a reasonable doubt that lowering elevated blood cholesterol levels will reduce the risk of heart attacks due to coronary heart disease. This has been demonstrated most conclusively in men with elevated blood cholesterol levels, but much evidence justifies the conclusion that similar protection will be afforded in women with elevated levels. ... Epidemiologic data and over a dozen clinical trials allow us to predict with reasonable assurance that such a measure will afford significant protection against coronary heart disease.

Their conclusion meant that *physicians could be reimbursed for testing for cholesterol,* and drug companies could sell "cholesterol lowering" drugs. This self-serving statement provided physicians with a simple treatment regimen that, not coincidentally, provided a huge financial windfall to the major drug companies.

In 2001, the National Heart, Lung and Blood Institute changed its tune. It published research which showed that a deficiency of linolenic acid (LNA, found in Omega-3 fatty acids) is the major cause of heart disease. What happened to cholesterol, all of a sudden? Does their latest announcement mean that they will now require physicians to test for LNA deficiency? They are still going for the simplistic answer. The fact is that Omega-3's alone won't eliminate your risk of heart disease any more than taking an anti-cholesterol pill would. *The real cause of heart disease is more complex than that.*

Trusting Your Own Instincts - Take Charge of Your Life

The medical community and the rest of the MIC are unlikely to change overnight. Its resistance to change, *its interests in profits and prestige,* has been with us for centuries. Unlike the patients of the 1500s, 1600s, and 1700s, *we have a choice. We can educate ourselves and take charge of our own health.* With the aid of the Internet and free access to the National Library of Medicine through PubMed (www.ncbi.nlm.nih.gov/entrez/query.fcgi), you and I have the same access to medical information as professional medical people.

You have a duty to yourself to take advantage of this unprecedented availability of information. It's your life, and your health that's at stake. It has the added benefit of setting you free of the need to run from doctor to doctor, spending a fortune on exams and medications. You'll discover that a healthy lifestyle which depends on wise choices based on accurate scientific knowledge will set you free from drugs and open up a more satisfying way of living.

Only *you* can decide to have a healthy, happy, drug-free life. *It really is up to you.* It may be time to tell the cholesterol terrorists to get lost — that you want to get healthy now, and not just have a low cholesterol value. You may no longer wish to waste your time getting tested for cholesterol, since it really does not appear to matter anyway — unless you were born with a genetic defect that causes sky-high cholesterol values. The key is to get the right nutrients into your body in the right amount at the right time from *fresh whole foods with pure water and exercise.* It is not as hard as you think. The next chapter will give you more information and an important quiz that will help you to prepare for this healthy new life.

– CHAPTER THREE –

Preparing For A
Fresh New Start

If the cholesterol terrorists were only guilty of putting out a flawed theory, something that affected only the world of scientific debate, there would be no reason to call them terrorists. The problem is they put out this theory to the public, under the guise of "experts," and their hope is that not just a few of us will fall for their claims—they actively push it down our throats, relentlessly marketing their products and suppressing the real science that we all deserve to know.

We do not have to sit by passively, letting the MIC and fear of malpractice lawyers dictate the terms of good heart health to us. We can take matters into our own hands, if we're willing to learn about the most precious possession any of us have: our health. That means understanding not only what's wrong with the cholesterol theory, but also what a better way of life–a healthier way of living–really looks like.

A Good Eggs-ample

As I said before, the cholesterol terrorists, through the MIC, oversimplify the whole issue of heart disease by attributing it almost entirely to the consumption of fats and cholesterol. Many people have taken the cholesterol theory to heart, cutting many fat- and cholesterol-bearing foods from their daily intake. Instead, they are buying everything labeled "fat-free" and "cholesterol-free" that they can find–but this is foolish.

For example, the one food that has perhaps gotten the worst rap from the cholesterol terrorists is the egg. Supposedly, the high-cholesterol content of the yolks is to blame, but there is no conclusive scientific evidence to justify the condemnation of this most nutritious of nature's foods. It's all guilt by association: eggs have cholesterol, so eggs must be bad.

So people don't eat eggs, switching to "no cholesterol" egg substitutes or at least switching to egg-white-only omelets and such. If eggs are so deadly, why is it that the Japanese, who have the lowest rate of heart disease in the world, are also the highest per-week consumers of eggs, averaging 6.3 per week? If you stick with the cholesterol terrorists' theory, this just doesn't make sense.

Eggs Represent Future Life
Scientific research, on the other hand, puts the picture into better perspective. Rather than focusing solely on the cholesterol in the egg, science shows just why this food, so life-sustaining for little chicks, is also nutrient-rich for us humans. A single whole egg contains 6 grams of high-quality protein, necessary for building muscles. The yolk, which the cholesterol terrorists would have you believe is so terrible, is in fact a great source of iron, zinc, the B vitamins (including folic acid), and vitamins D and E. How about choline? This nutrient is important for preventing memory loss, and eggs are by far the richest natural source of choline: two eggs provide 50 percent of the RDA.

If you listen to the cholesterol terrorists, you'll cut eggs out of your diet. That means you will cut out all these other important nutrients as well and all because of the false claim, pushed by the MIC, that cholesterol is the be-all and end-all of heart disease. According to the latest scientific studies, one of which involved 38,000 men and 80,000 women over a 20-year period, there was absolutely no increase in risk if participants ate just 1 egg per week or had an egg every day. In the Ireland-Boston Heart Study, researchers looked at two populations: 600 Boston men of Irish descent aged 30 to 60, who had lived in America for at least 10 years, and compared them to their brothers, who had never left the Old Country. The Boston population ate about half as many eggs, on average, as their Irish counterparts, who consumed about 14 per week. The Irish brothers had lower blood cholesterol levels, and when measured by other indicators, their hearts seemed in noticeably better health than the American participants in the study.

Eggs provide a great example of how deeply flawed the cholesterol theory really is. If it were true, you would expect the Irish brothers in the study just mentioned to be in bad shape, at least with regard to heart disease. In fact the opposite is true—and that makes sense if you recognize that there are lots of factors, not just one or two, which make for good heart health. For example, the Irish brothers appear to have lived a more physically active lifestyle, so exercise probably had an effect.

Eggs Are Important

Why is this information about eggs so important? One very important reason is that more and more people are turning to vegetarianism in their quest for health. For vegetarians, it is difficult to get substantial amounts of Omega-3 fatty acids into their diets (more on Omega-3s later in the book). If their vegetarian regimen permits eggs, this possible deficiency can be easily overcome, because each egg can contain from 200 to 500 milligrams of Omega-3s and some of it is long chain Omega-3 like fish.

The Secret Downside of Anti-Cholesterol Drugs

The pharmaceutical industry is careful in what they say about their products. They are willing to imply that buying their drugs will improve your heart health, but if you look closely at their literature and web sites, and read all the tiny print, you're in for a big surprise. Lipitor®, for example, is the best-selling anti-cholesterol drug on the market today, and I invite you to check out the manufacturer's web page for the product at www.lipitor.com/risk/cholesterolandheartdisease.asp. After making the expected connection between cholesterol build-up and heart disease, complete with graphics, Lipitor® is forced by their lawyers or the FDA to make the following statement: "Lipitor® has not been shown to prevent heart disease or heart attacks."

The Dark Side of Lipitor®

Well, if it doesn't prevent heart disease or heart attacks, then why take it, especially when you read the even smaller print that details the problems with the drug? For example, Lipitor's own website and ads admit that people with liver problems and nursing or pregnant women (and women who might become pregnant) should not take their drug. In addition, all cholesterol-lowering drugs have the potential to cause impotence in men. Why? Because the hormones that govern the sex drive are themselves formed from cholesterol. If you lower your cholesterol too far, you don't make the hormones!

Even so, for a drug that even the manufacturer says doesn't work to prevent heart disease, Lipitor® rakes in something like $2 billion per year for its patent holders. You can probably bet that we wouldn't even get the small-print warnings that the product doesn't prevent heart disease if it weren't for FDA regulations. The question is, if the drug doesn't improve our heart health, why are so many of us buying it? The simple answer is that most of us don't really understand our bodies and what they need, so we're easy prey for the MIC's promises of "quick fixes."

There Are No Quick Fixes

Quick fixes can be dangerous. That's what Drs. T. Newman and S. Hulley, researchers at the Department of Laboratory Medicine, University of California at San Francisco discovered. Their research showed that anti-cholesterol drugs were linked to increased cancers. Their findings were so chilling that they offered the following conclusion, in a report published in the January 1996 issue of the *Journal of the American Medical Association*: "The results of experiments... suggest that lipid-lowering [anti-cholesterol] drug treatment... should be avoided except in patients at high short-term risk of coronary heart disease." Good advice, since even without the increased risk of cancer, the drugs simply don't seem to work. Drs. M. F. Muldoon, S. B. Manuck, and K. A.

Matthews of the Department of Medicine at the University of Pittsburgh concur. In their 1990 article, they reported "the failure of cholesterol lowering drugs to affect overall survival justifies a more cautious appraisal of the probable benefits of lowering cholesterol in the general population.

How to Plug an Artery

That's why I say the first thing you need to do is get a good basic understanding about heart disease and the factors that contribute to it. The basic mechanism that leads to cardiovascular disease, including heart attacks, is fairly easy to understand. Even the cholesterol terrorists get a part of it right: step one on the road to a heart attack is plugging up your arteries. If your eating habits are like those of many Americans, you're probably well on your way to doing just that.

Plugging an artery *does* take some effort; however, given the availability of heart-stopping foods at every corner store, it isn't all that hard. You start by eating a lot of the following things:

- Sugar that is quickly converted to saturated fat in the body

- Fat from an animal that becomes loaded with free radicals during grilling, and is high in saturated fat loaded with hormones

- Bleached white flour products that contain few nutrients, but lots of oxidized compounds that enter into the bloodstream very quickly

● Polyunsaturated fat that can easily become oxidized.

After eating this type of diet, the Omega-6 fat causes the cells in the lining of the artery (the endothelium) to become inflamed. Free radicals from rancid fat molecules attack the lining of the arteries. The arteries become very inflamed and very irritated by the free radicals that become attached to it, ultimately eating a hole into the arterial wall. Meanwhile, the excess sugar you're consuming results in the formation of insulin molecules, which eat away at the hole in the artery, enlarging it. Soon you have a hole big enough to permit leakage: you're now dealing with internal bleeding! What's the body to do?

The body wants to heal itself. It sends in platelets and white blood cells to patch the hole, but the free radicals and insulin are right there, ripping off the patch as quickly as the white blood cells can make it. Soon the body tries a new tactic: it knows that saturated fat molecules are big and sticky, and it tries using them to plug the hole. Next thing you know, you've got plaque build-up and a badly plugged artery.

Notice in all of this, the primary causes—the Omega-6s, for example, and the free radicals and excess insulin—can't be taken out of the equation by cutting out cholesterol. The problem is too complex. That means that the cholesterol theory is too deeply flawed to address it.

The Disintegration of the Cholesterol Theory

While few within the MIC have been willing to acknowledge the flaws in their cholesterol theory, there has been great interest in the research community for a more complete understanding of the causes of heart disease. The research, which you'll read in greater detail in the chapters to come, has finally begun to have an effect! For example, 17 years ago the Heart, Lung, and Blood Institute convened the Cholesterol Consensus Conference, in effect officially placing its prestige and authority behind the cholesterol theory. Sixteen years later, in the November 2001 issue of the *American Journal of Clinical Nutrition*, this same organization reversed itself completely, acknowledging the important role that alpha linolenic acid (the plant-based version of Omega-3 fatty acid, found in abundance in flax seeds) plays in reducing the risk of heart disease. Nice to see the rest of the world is finally catching up with what some of us have been saying for years: fresh, whole-grain foods, rich in Omega-3, are key to living a heart healthy lifestyle!

Let's not commit the same mistake that the cholesterol terrorists made in settling for a simplistic answer to a complex problem. Omega-3s are important, but so are fiber, pure water, regular exercise, B vitamins, antioxidants, and trace minerals. Research has shown that all together, these factors can reduce your risk of heart disease by as much as 70 percent. Reducing fat and cholesterol reduces your risk of heart disease a *further 10 percent!!!*

What is WE-FOBAM

To truly break free of the overly simplistic, pseudo-solution offered by the cholesterol terrorists, then, you need to take a whole new look at the foods you eat. Since most people don't have a degree in nutrition, this can seem pretty daunting. That's where this book comes in. I have developed a comprehensive approach to heart-healthy living, a Maximum Quality of Life Plan, which is designed to make it easier for you to take charge of your health. Remember, heart health is dependent on many factors, not just one, so the program is multifaceted. To help yourself remember all of its elements, think in terms of this acronym: WE-FOBAM. Here's what it stands for:

W = *Water, essential for life*

E = *Exercise, to keep fit and strong*

F = *Fiber, nature's greatest cleaning aid*

O = *Omega-3s, the fatty acids that work miracles*

B = *B-vitamins, including folic acid*

A = *Antioxidants, to wipe out nasty free radicals*

M = *Minerals, essential building blocks of health*

Note that, with regard to foods, this diet differs substantially from the diet traditionally recommended by the American Heart Association, which was far too focused on the whole low-cholesterol issue. The good news is that the AHA has recently rethought its commitment to the cholesterol terrorists and in November of 2002, has officially altered its dietary recommendations to include an acknowledgement of the importance of Omega-3s (see Chapter 7 for more details).

By including all of the WE-FOBAM factors in your lifestyle and diet, you can achieve what all of the anti-cholesterol theorists have failed to do: substantially reduce your risk of heart disease. What's more, this program has positive effects for lots of other physical conditions that may have damaged the quality of your life, including joint pain from arthritis!

Drugs Versus WE-FOBAM

By adopting the WE-FOBAM lifestyle, you increase your consumption of all these important nutrients. At the same time, you reduce your consumption of all those elements that contribute to heart disease: highly processed foods for the most part. By doing so you easily and naturally improve your heart health. As an added benefit, you save yourself a lot of money. After all, the drugs that loom large in the MIC's cholesterol theory cost a fortune and have many nasty side effects. In the end you're still likely to be looking at a bypass operation or other hospital intervention because the drugs simply have no effect on reducing your risk of heart disease.

In the majority of trials comparing cholesterol-lowering drugs with some parts of a good, whole-foods approach such as the WE-FOBAM program, the drugs come out the losers. In most cases they compared the drugs with people on a very sub-optimal diet. In the next seven chapters, we will present each element of the WE-FOBAM approach in detail, explaining just what the latest research tells us about their effects. In addition, we offer advice on how you can most easily maximize each element in your own life.

Before we get started, here are a series of self-tests that will let you take stock of just how your current diet and lifestyle stacks up. When you're through, you will have a better idea of where you're deficient in necessary nutrients and be able to tailor your own program to meet your particular needs. So, get your pencils sharpened and... Ready, Set, Go!

What is Your Vitality Score

Symptoms of Omega-3 Deficiency

Place a 1, 2, 3, or 4 next to all signs or symptoms

1 = seldom; 2 = mild; 3 = moderate; 4 = severe

_____ Dry skin
_____ Dry, rough patches on elbows
_____ Dry, dull hair
_____ Insatiable thirst
_____ Bumps or skin like a chicken
_____ Soft or brittle nails
_____ Uncontrollable allergies
_____ Difficulty with attention or focus
_____ Hyperactivity
_____ Aggression or hostility
_____ Irritability
_____ Depression
_____ Learning difficulty
_____ Poor memory
_____ Reading difficulty
_____ Heart rhythm problems
_____ High cholesterol
_____ Joint Inflammation
_____ Fatigue
_____ Heart disease
_____ Arthritis
_____ Diabetes

_____ **Total Points**

Less than 8 = Good
8 to 15   = Likely evidence of Omega-3 deficiency;
                need to take 1000 Omega-3 from flax
                per day
15 to 20   = Strong evidence of Omega-3 deficiency;
                need to take 3000 mg. Omega-3 from
                flax per day
20 or more = Need to take 1000 mg DHA daily, plus
                5000 mg. Omega-3 from flax per day

Trans Fatty Acid Score

Place a 1, 2, 3, or 4 next to each question based on which best describes your dietary intake of the following foods.

0 = never; 1 = less than once per month; 2 = once a month; 3. = daily use

_____ French fries
_____ Chicken nuggets
_____ Potato chips
_____ Corn or tortilla chips
_____ Deep fried fish or chicken or steak
_____ Butter
_____ Cheese
_____ Milk
_____ Donuts
_____ Pastries
_____ Margarine
_____ Mayonnaise
_____ Cake
_____ Cookies
_____ White bread
_____ Soft, brown breads (fake whole wheat)
_____ Shortening
_____ Puffed cheese snacks
_____ **Total Points**

Less than 5 = Great
5 to 12   = Better watch out
12 or more = Better negotiate a reduced cost funeral at the local morgue

Exercise Score

Seldom exercise	= 0
Walks 2 to 5 blocks weekly	= 1
Walks 2 to 5 blocks daily	= 2
Walks 1 to 3 miles per week	= 3
Walks 3 to 5 miles per week	= 5
Jogs 3 to 5 miles weekly	= 5
Jogs more than 5 miles weekly	= 8

Total Points _____

Omega-3 Score

Place a 1, 2, 3, or 4 next to each question based on which best describes your dietary intake of the following foods.

---

0 = never; 1 = once per month; 2 = twice a month; 3 = weekly; 4 = twice a week; 5 = daily

---

_____ Salmon
_____ Mackerel
_____ Herring
_____ Sardines
_____ Anchovies
_____ Tuna
_____ Flax fed eggs
_____ Stabilized, fortified flax drink mix
          (like Ultra Omega Balance or
          Sweet to the Heart)
_____ Freshly squeezed fruits and vegetables
_____ Breads containing flax
_____ Flax cereals
_____ Flax bagels
_____ Walnuts
_____ Pumpkin seeds
_____ Brazil nuts
_____ Pecans
_____ Almonds or almond butter
_____ Extra virgin olive oil
_____ Canola oil
_____ Dark green leafy vegetables
_____ Trans fat free spreads

_____ **Total Points**

Less than 5 = Far too little Omega-3 to prevent a hear attack, diabetes or arthritis

5 to 10   = Modest intake

10 to 30   = Will probably have average health

30 or more = Will probably have superior health.
             **May die from swimming in the ocean
             at age 96 like my hero Paul Bragg.**

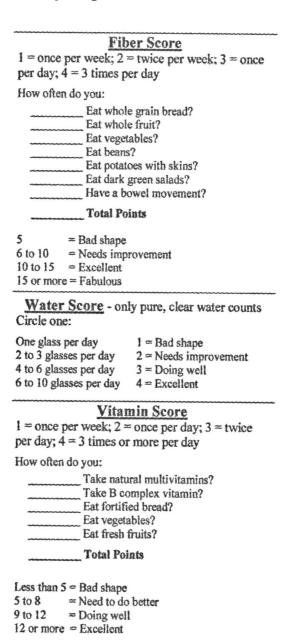

Fiber Score

1 = once per week; 2 = twice per week; 3 = once per day; 4 = 3 times per day

How often do you:

_____ Eat whole grain bread?
_____ Eat whole fruit?
_____ Eat vegetables?
_____ Eat beans?
_____ Eat potatoes with skins?
_____ Eat dark green salads?
_____ Have a bowel movement?

_____ **Total Points**

5   = Bad shape
6 to 10   = Needs improvement
10 to 15   = Excellent
15 or more   = Fabulous

Water Score - only pure, clear water counts

Circle one:

One glass per day	1 = Bad shape
2 to 3 glasses per day	2 = Needs improvement
4 to 6 glasses per day	3 = Doing well
6 to 10 glasses per day	4 = Excellent

Vitamin Score

1 = once per week; 2 = once per day; 3 = twice per day; 4 = 3 times or more per day

How often do you:

_____ Take natural multivitamins?
_____ Take B complex vitamin?
_____ Eat fortified bread?
_____ Eat vegetables?
_____ Eat fresh fruits?

_____ **Total Points**

Less than 5 = Bad shape
5 to 8   = Need to do better
9 to 12   = Doing well
12 or more   = Excellent

*This quiz has been modified from Michael Schmidt's book *Brain Building Nutrition,* which I highly recommend.

Now that you've taken stock, are you ready to learn more? Let's move on to Chapter 4 and begin with the most basic element of a healthy lifestyle: plain old, pure water.

CHAPTER FOUR

Water, Water Everywhere...

Let's begin with one of the most basic elements of life, the first letter in our WE-FOBAM acronym: Water. Most people take water for granted—after all, it contains no "nutritional value": no vitamins or minerals. Water, like oxygen, is essential to life. For optimal health, an adequate supply of water is as important as protein, carbohydrates, fats, vitamins, and minerals. You might even say that it's more important: you can live for a week or more without proteins, carbohydrates, and fats, but you can only live a few days without water. Here are a few facts about water that you might find surprising:

• Seventy-five percent of Americans are chronically dehydrated, and half the world population is likely to be dehydrated.

• The thirst mechanism in 37 percent of Americans is so weak that it is frequently mistaken for hunger pangs instead.

• Even mild dehydration will slow down metabolism as much as 3 percent!

• In a University of Washington study, one glass of water shuts down midnight hunger pains in almost 100 percent of dieters. Odds are, it will work for you!

• There is preliminary research that indicates drinking 8 to 10 8-ounce glasses of water a day could significantly ease back and joint pain for up to 80 percent of sufferers.

• Lack of water is the NUMBER ONE trigger of daytime fatigue!

• A mere 2 percent drop in body water can trigger fuzzy short-term memory, trouble with basic math, and difficulty focusing on the computer or reading printed material.

• By drinking a mere 5 glasses of water each day, you decrease the risk of breast cancer by 79 percent and you are 50 percent less likely to develop bladder cancer and 50% less likely to die of heart disease.

The Life-Giving Role of Water

We need water for every major bodily function: temperature control, digestion, and waste and toxin removal. Overall, about 55 to 60 percent of your body is made up of water, although the percentage varies greatly depending on the organ or system you're looking at. For example, your bones are just 25 percent water, but your brain is 76 percent water and your lungs are a whopping 90 percent—even more than your body's most familiar fluid, blood, which weighs in at 82 percent water. Your brain is your body's most urgent water consumer: it is the first organ to suffer the ill-effects of even minor dehydration, and the first to get water after a period of deprivation, because it is so necessary to prioritizing the delivery and use of water to the rest of your body.

Everything you do affects the water content of your body. For example, you lose two cups of water every day, just by breathing. You lose another two cups invisibly, through normal perspiration as your body strives to regulate its internal temperature. You lose a full six cups every day through the elimination of bodily wastes. Keeping your body's water content in balance is important: your tissues need to retain enough to stay properly hydrated even though you're losing significant amounts of it with every action–even every breath–you take.

Staying in Balance

Your body's ability to retain this life-sustaining substance in its tissues can be affected by a wide range of factors. Physical exertion, stress, and the consumption of alcohol and caffeine speed up the removal of water from your system. Even the weather can have an impact: you perspire far more on very hot days. Salts and carbohydrates, on the other hand, cause your body to retain more water than it normally needs, which is why these items can sometimes make you feel uncomfortable, a condition commonly called "bloating."

To keep your body in balance, you need to consume adequate supplies of water throughout the day. This is called rehydration: the replacement of water that has been lost through elimination and perspiration. Most of the foods and beverages you consume contain at least some water, but some are more efficient sources than others, and some will even cause your body to lose water faster than normal. Alcoholic and caffeinated beverages are two major offenders in this regard. Your best choice is the simplest one: drink lots of plain water every day.

What Does The Science Say

Recent scientific research is beginning to show just how important it is to keep your body adequately hydrated, especially when it comes to maintaining a heart-healthy lifestyle. An amazing study published in the May 2002 issue of the *American Journal of Epidemiology* shows that drinking 5 glasses of water each day cuts the risk of having a heart attack by 54 percent in men and 41 percent in women. The research, known as the Adventist Health Study, monitored 20,000 people for a period of six years. The study participants were all people who were at low risk of heart disease–in other words, they did not have lifestyle or family issues that made them highly likely to suffer from the disease. With results like this for a relatively low-risk group, imagine how much better the results would be for people at high risk of heart disease.

To really appreciate the value of water in lowering your risk for heart disease, let's consider how simply increasing your intake of water stacks up against other steps you could take. For example, we've all heard about how taking an aspirin a day is supposed to reduce your risk of heart disease, and then there are the more recent announcements about the benefit of moderate red wine consumption. Well, the benefit from increasing your water intake was found to be greater than either of these. In fact, drinking water seems to confer as much benefit to heart health as stopping smoking!

It is important to remember, however, that all fluids are not created equal. Water provides proven benefits, but other fluids, like soda pop, actually increase the risk of having a heart attack by 247 percent in women and 146 percent in men. The simple solution is to focus on fresh, clean water. This is far better than any drug ever tested.

An Extraordinary Study

The health benefits of water have been documented in an extraordinary book called *Your Body's Many Cries for Water*, written by an Iranian physician named Feyedoon Batmanghelidj. Batmanghelidj was held as a political prisoner in Iran, and while in prison he attempted to ease the suffering of his fellow inmates. As a prisoner, however, he had no access to medicines–all he had was water. The results he achieved by offering only water were astounding. His book tells an astounding story, but it is marred by the fact that he used highly clinical language, making it difficult for nonspecialist readers to understand.

Says Dr. Batmanghelidj: "If we begin to appreciate that for the process of digestion of food, water is the most essential ingredient, most of the battle is won. If we give the necessary water to the body before we eat food, all the battle against cholesterol formation in the blood vessels will be won."

How much is enough? Remember, dehydration by as little as 2 percent of your body weight can result in impaired physiological and performance responses. Dr. S. M. Kleiner, at the University of Washington, recommends 12 cups of fluid per day for the average sedentary adult man and 9 cups of fluid a day for the average sedentary adult woman. Maintaining proper hydration can offer benefits that go far beyond keeping your heart healthy. It can reduce your risk of urinary stone disease and cancers of the breast, colon and urinary tract. It helps reduce the incidence of childhood and adolescent obesity. It can reduce the risk of mitral valve prolapse, in which the little flaps that separate the chambers of your heart from one another fail to open and close properly, disturbing or halting the regular flow of blood through that organ. It can improve your salivary gland function. In other words, getting an adequate daily supply of water has important implications for your overall health.

Considerations Regarding the Water You Drink

Remember what I said earlier in this chapter, "What you drink is as important as getting enough to drink." Some fluids act as diuretics–they speed the elimination of water from the body, which is the exact opposite of what we're hoping to achieve! Even if you consume a large volume of fluids, if they have a diuretic property you can still be dehydrated. Use the following list as a guide:

Hydrating Fluids and Foods	Dehydrating Fluids (diuretic)
Water (plain, sparkling, or mineral)	Alcoholic beverages
Juice	Caffeinated beverages including:
Herbal teas	Coffee
Non-caffeinated drinks/sports drinks/ sodas	Tea
Non-alcoholic beverages	Sodas with caffeine
Vegetables	Water with added caffeine
Fruits	
Soups	

The best choice of all is fresh, clean water. Unfortunately, most of us don't have a clear mountain spring nearby. Tap water may have chemical additives (such as fluoride or chlorine), which can give it an unappealing taste or smell. Bottled water, on the other hand, generally avoids these "cosmetic" issues, but believe it or not, it is not necessarily more pure than the water that comes out of your tap and does have a lot less chlorine. That's because your tap water is tested by your local municipality for purity, whereas bottled water is not. In the end, you might just decide to opt for filtering your own tap water, which should remove any unpleasant odors or taste.

Getting Enough

Because we tend to take water for granted, many of us are surprised to discover that we are not getting anywhere near enough of it every day. Remember the quiz you took at the end of the last chapter? If you scored low for water consumption, it's time to take action. Fortunately, there are some very simple ways that you can easily increase the amount of water you drink each day. Here are just a few:

• Get portable water bottles and carry them with you wherever you go. It's easy today, since 'drinking cap' water bottles are found in virtually every convenience store and gas station.

• While you're at it, recycle those purchased bottles–refill them at home with filtered tap water and keep a good store of them in the refrigerator.

• Instead of soda, coffee, or tea, order water with your meals in restaurants. Even fast-food places offer a bottled water option.

• Keep one of your refilled water bottles with you when watching TV. Sipping cool water will keep you from reaching for the high fat, high salt snack foods.

• For you smokers who are trying to quit: keep bottled water with you to sip whenever a craving hits.

• Drink two glasses of water before every meal. This will help you eat less and aid digestion.

• Measure out the amount you want to drink in a day into a pitcher. It will remind you of your commitment and help you keep track of your intake.

How much water is the right amount for you? According to S. M. Kleiner of the Nutritional Sciences Program, University of Washington, Seattle, the average sedentary adult male should be getting at least 96 ounces (12 cups) of fluids each day. For women the volume is a little lower: 72 ounces (9 cups). While water is preferable, fluids can also include noncaffeinated beverages (nonalcoholic, please) and soups. About 4 cups, or 32 ounces, of the total daily intake is taken care of by the water that is contained in the foods you eat.

Bottom line, you need water. Drink lots of it; enjoy it. Whether you choose bottled water or tap, your body will thank you.

Before you go overboard, keep in mind that it is possible to drink too much water. Too much water can result in water intoxication. This kind of problem can happen with marathon runners and athletes who consume massive amounts of water before a big event or obsessive/compulsive people who don't know when to stop. By the way, if you've taken steps to increase your water consumption but you don't seem to be able to allay your thirst, take notice. Chronic thirst is one of the symptoms of diabetes. Talk to your doctor–you may be well advised to get a full work-up.

CHAPTER FIVE

Exercise

The second element of the WE-FOBAM program is an obvious one, but one that too many of us neglect in our daily lives. That's right, I'm talking about exercise. One of the reasons that the MIC is so successful in selling its cholesterol theory of heart disease is that we, as a nation, are all too willing to turn to pills and fads in order to avoid increasing our daily activity rate. Exercise is fundamental to good heart health–in fact, it's fundamental to all aspects of your general health and well-being.

Fitness and Health

You have 640 muscles in your body. This number includes the big muscles that let you move your legs and the little ones that let you crook your pinky finger. What most people don't recognize is that the word "muscle" includes more than the familiar abs, triceps, and biceps–your organs are muscles too! Along with your brain, your heart is perhaps the most important muscle in your body! Exercise keeps your heart healthy so that it can do its work for the rest of your body.

If you are like the majority of adult Americans, however, it's probably not a good idea for you to rush right out to start a high-intensity exercise program this very minute. As we get older, most of us ease up on the natural activity levels that were so easy to maintain when we were younger. On top of this, most of us have indulged in less than optimal diets—eating foods high in saturated fats, salts, sugars, and so forth. As a result, it is highly probable that, like many adult Americans, your arteries have become filled with sludge over the years. If you got up right now and started exercising strenuously, you'd increase the rate of blood flow through your body, which would get that sludge circulating right along with it. This is not a result that you particularly want to achieve.

In addition, a poor diet may have left you carrying around extra weight. If so, you are not alone–obesity in adults and children is at an epidemic level these days. Exercise can help you eliminate that extra weight, but you have to be careful. You can do yourself great harm if you started a strenuous exercise program without changing the quality of your diet. Exercise is only one component of a larger lifestyle change: to receive the benefits, you need to make sure that the other components are in place, too.

What The Science Says

Pretty much everybody agrees on the value of exercise, even if we are individually reluctant to do it often enough. It is helpful to review some of the most recent research results: you might even find them inspiring enough to prompt you to get a little more activity into your days! Here's a quick sampling of what the scientists have been saying lately.

Read on about some results of recent scientific studies on the benefits of exercise.

• In the January 2001 issue of the *Annual of*

Internal Medicine, a study conducted by a team of Harvard researchers for the Harvard School of Public Health found that vigorous exercise for 2 to 4 hours per week reduced the risk of heart disease by 18 percent. Just walking for 1-2 hours per week was almost as good, giving a risk reduction of 15 percent. Doubling their walking time per week (2 to 4 hours) more than doubled the risk reduction–to 37%!

• In May 2001, in the *Ugeskr Laeger,* a Danish team published their findings after a 17-year-long study of 4,658 men from ages 20 to 79 years. They found that study participants who jogged regularly had a significantly lower mortality rate than non-joggers. We can't give jogging all the credit for this study's findings: other lifestyle factors may also have contributed to the results.

• A 1994 study conducted at the Veterans Affairs Medical Center in Sepulveda, CA, included both men and women. It found that women who exercised the most lived the longest. Another study by the same research facility looked specifically at the effects of exercise on diabetic women. They found that increased physical activity (including regular walking) is associated with a substantially reduced risk for cardiovascular events.

• A study published in the February 1993 issue of the *New England Journal of Medicine* also corroborated the fact that increased physical activity can significantly extend your lifespan.

• In the October 1992 issue of the *Journal of the American Medical Association,* Harvard College alumni were monitored to determine the impacts of a healthier lifestyle, with specific reference to the following four factors: beginning a moderately vigorous sports activity, quitting smoking, maintaining normal blood pressure, and avoiding obesity. Every one of these factors was individually associated with lower rates of death, including coronary heart disease.

Your Body as a Car

If exercise is so important, you may be surprised that I suggest you wait a bit before really getting into an exercise regimen, especially if you've been indulging in poor eating habits up to now. To understand why I say this, think of your body as a car. Years of low-quality eating habits have built up sludge in the fuel system, and the extra weight you've put on is like a thousand-pound bag of sand stuffed into the trunk. When you start the car up–that is, when you begin an exercise program–the sandbag will surely slow it down, and the sludge will make the engine overheat and burn up.

To continue our car analogy, years of poor nutrition have also damaged essential parts. When you are eating poor foods, your organs are not receiving the nutrition they need to function at top capacity. Your engine doesn't get enough fuel (poor blood flow), and your tires are under inflated (inadequate respiratory function). No car in that condition can travel far before it breaks down, right? The same is true for your body.

Most heart disease is caused by a lack of vital nutrients in the body's tissues. The deficiencies cause problems even before you develop full-blown heart disease, just as a car with a faulty fuel delivery system will start acting up long before it had its final breakdown on the highway. If you start an exercise program without first making sure that you've corrected these deficiencies, it's a little like taking your car out for a cross-country race without checking the fuel, oil, and water–you're just asking for a major breakdown once you're on the road.

Putting First Things First

Before you start a serious exercise program, it's best to clean up your diet. With nutrient-rich blood flowing through your arteries, you'll begin to clear some of the sludge out of your system, and your body will begin to heal itself. The benefits are noticeable almost at once: you start feeling better, more energetic, more physically strong. Because your body has the chance to begin healing itself before you "hit the road," you can avoid most of the physical discomfort that we associate with starting a new exercise program.

We highly recommend that you follow the WE-FOBAM diet for at least 6 weeks before you do any strenuous exercise. Exercise is good for your health, but it can cause a lot of stress on your heart, lungs, and arteries if they're plugged up and weak from years of poor nutrition and sedentary living. That's not to say that you should be a couch-potato during that first 6 weeks. In fact, you can start gentle, non-strenuous walking right at the beginning of your diet change. The important thing is to pay attention to what your body tells you. Listen to your heart, and if you feel any discomfort, give your system a chance to get healthy, then you can give it good robust workouts to keep it in good shape.

Aerobic and Anaerobic Exercise

There are two types of exercise, aerobic and anaerobic, and each one provides a different type of benefit. Both are important to incorporate into your lifestyle.

Aerobic (oxygen burning) exercise strengthens your heart, lungs and bones, improves intestinal function, improves mental outlook, and allows you to eat more without gaining weight. You may live a longer, healthier life because it improves your body's usage of oxygen. Aerobic exercise includes walking, running, jogging, biking, or any other activity that requires you to increase your heart rate substantially.

Anaerobic (non-oxygen burning) exercise focuses on particular muscle masses, and serves to strengthen and build up actual muscle tissue, primarily by the repeated flex and contraction of the muscles. The anaerobic exercise most folks recognize is weight lifting. Stronger, denser muscles have greater strength, giving you increased endurance and an improved metabolism. Those are great results!

Both aerobic and anaerobic exercises have an important place in a healthy overall lifestyle. The benefits include improved stamina, more efficient oxygen use, and improved respiration and circulation. They both con-

tribute to raising your metabolism as well–which is important for weight control.

Dieting Versus Exercise

With all the recent news about the epidemic of obesity in America, we're all a lot more conscious of our
weight. Unfortunately for lots of people, this means getting involved in fad diets instead of really learning about
their bodies' nutritional needs. The MIC is right there,
ready and waiting to take advantage of the trend: Weight
reduction programs abound. The problem is that most of
the commercial weight-loss programs and "get thin quick"
diets focus on weight-loss, not overall health. What's
worse, most of them are unsuccessful even in their primary goal of weight loss: statistics show that most dieters
regain the weight they've lost–and more–within a year!

Why does this happen? The answer lies deep in the
brain, in an organ known as the hypothalamus. You can
think of the hypothalamus as the body's commander,
charged with the responsibility of keeping everything in
balance. It gets its instructions mostly from our genes,
and among its instructions is our metabolic setting, which
regulates the rate with which the body burns its fuel: the
calories we eat. This setting is relatively resistant to
change; otherwise, our weight would fluctuate wildly
every time we ate more or less, exercised more or less,
and hydrated our bodies more or less.

The problem that dieters run into when they're trying to lose weight comes from the hypothalamus's resistance to change. When you cut back on the calories you
consume, the hypothalamus starts worrying about the

future, and stores some of them as fat for future use. You have to cut back pretty far–or burn calories significantly faster–to actually start to see the pounds begin to drop away. Then, after all that work, when you finally reach your dieting goal and go back to your normal eating patterns, the hypothalamus swings into action to bring you back to the weight it is programmed to view as "normal." Unfortunately, that's usually the weight you were at before you went on the diet.

The secret to lasting weight loss is not found in dieting. The secret is in something called your "set point." This is the setting that your hypothalamus considers to be proper for your body, the weight that your body will constantly strive to return to, even after you've dieted away several pounds. To successfully achieve a healthy weight, you have to alter that setting, in effect reprogramming your hypothalamus.

There are two ways to alter the hypothalamic set point for your appetite and weight. The first, and by far the worst, is to try to change it by taking stimulant drugs. These artificially increase your metabolic rate, causing you to burn calories faster and confusing your hypothalamus into neglecting its job. These drugs can cause serious damage to your system, as anyone who takes the time to read the small print on the packaging will learn. Why run these risks if there's a healthier, simpler way?

That healthy option is to pay attention to the nutrients you consume–in other words, learn to eat healthy–and to increase your daily activity levels. In the upcoming chapters you'll learn more about the "eating healthy" part of this equation. For now it's only important to know that a healthy diet omits artificial flavorings and other additives, and is rich in all the essential nutrients that your present diet quite probably lacks.

Before we leave the subject of commercial diets, however, there's one more important point to make. Some of these diets have been around for years, and you probably know several people who claim that they've had great success. Because the diets, and the dieters who follow them, focus only on weight loss, they fail to notice the potential dangers that these diets represent. For example, there's the famous Atkins Diet, developed by Dr. Robert Atkins, which relies on a high-protein, low-cholesterol approach to weight loss. The problem with this one is that the high protein content of the diet can do great harm to the kidneys and liver, which are forced to work overtime to detoxify the body of all that extra protein. It has a history of actually contributing to heart trouble–as Dr. Atkins experienced himself in March of 2002, when he developed heart problems. The focus on simple weight loss is misplaced. What good does it do to lose weight and end up with heart disease? All that does for you is to end up with a lighter casket at your funeral.

While I strongly suggest that you give the WE-FOBAM program a try, there are other alternatives out there that are less likely to cause the kinds of problems associated with dieting. Among the better programs are those that, like Weight Watchers, provide group support. Most importantly, pick a group that bases its dietary recommendations on the amount of fiber, fats, and nutrients you're consuming, and not just on counting calories.

Stress Control

If you are like many other people when you're feeling particularly stressed, you probably think that your best bet is to withdraw–to crash onto the sofa or crawl into bed and just "cool out." In fact, that's the exact opposite of what you need. Activity, whether it is formal exercise in the gym or informal exercise like taking a long walk or going for a bike ride, is a great stress reliever. Getting too little exercise actually contributes to your stress level.

Here's how it works. Stress causes many problems for the healthy functioning of your body. For example, when you're stressed your muscles grow tense, causing strain to the tissues; the chemical "fallout" from accumulated adrenaline output become toxins in your system (your body produces excess adrenaline to cope with stress); and high stress can seriously disrupt your ability to maintain your normal sleep schedule, leaving you exhausted. Exercise relieves many of these problems. Exercise reduces the muscle tension caused by stress, and by increasing your blood flow it helps cleanse your system of the toxic build-up of adrenaline and its by-products. By providing your body with a healthy dose of activity, exercise helps ensure that you'll get a good night's sleep. In addition, physical activity causes your body to release endorphins, a type of hormone that contributes to a sense of well being. In fact, the mental benefits are often more immediate and gratifying than the long-term physical benefits. One woman I know puts it this way: "I exercise for my mind, and my body goes along."

Remember that exercise is not only about physical exertion. Many exercise programs, such as those based on yoga techniques, also include an emphasis on meditation, and this is a great way to reduce stress. So is spending time with people you love–so get out there and give as many hugs as you can! Take stock of your life and see where you can reduce your stress: find work you enjoy doing, or if you can't change your job, find ways to make it less stressful.

Reduce the Effects of Aging

Finally, exercise helps to reduce the negative effects associated with aging. As we advance in years, our susceptibility to serious disease–from heart disease to diabetes to cancer–increases. We also begin to notice a reduction in physical mobility and in energy. Many of us experience weight gain. The skin loses some of its youthful glow and elasticity. With all these changes, many of us lose confidence and self esteem.

Exercise counteracts many of these effects. Properly done, with warm-up and cool-down stretches, exercise helps to keep your body limber and flexible. It helps you manage that "middle-age" weight gain and keep you looking fit and trim. It improves your circulation and elimination processes, so that your body remains cleared of toxins that would otherwise build up in your system. Those endorphins released by physical activity also contribute an important anti-aging effect: they make you feel good about yourself, which naturally makes you look better, too.

Before we leave the subject of the anti-aging benefits of exercise, however, there's one final effect that must be mentioned. Any exercise, whether it's a workout in the gym or a long walk in the country, is made more effective when it is accompanied by proper deep-breathing techniques. You want to use your full lung capacity, not just the 10 percent that most people use. In fact, there's a wonderful program developed by Jill R. Johnson, called *Oxycise!*, available on videotape. It is available in most major video stores.

Reducing the Risk of Heart Disease

Most people think of exercise only in the context of weight loss, but these days we're beginning to truly understand that becoming fit is more important than becoming lean, and this is especially true if you are at risk of heart disease. In fact, even if you are overweight, you can reduce your chances of a heart attack by 50 percent if you exercise regularly. That's what the Cooper Aerobics Center discovered: "fit but fat" people have a lower risk of heart disease than lean-bodied people who don't make regular activity a part of their daily routine. The health benefits of keeping fit don't stop with your heart: it also reduces your chances of dying from cancer, diabetes, arthritis, and other chronic diseases–even if you smoke. So even if you can't seem to drop those extra pounds, don't think that exercise is a waste of time.

Cycling and Surgery Have Similar Effect*

Among people with chest pain because of clogged heart arteries, regular exercise on a stationary bike reduced symptoms better than surgery did, a team of German physicians has found in a small study.

After a year, just 6 of the 51 of the patients in the study who exercised had either died or gone back to the hospital for additional procedures, while 15 of the 50 patients who had angioplasty had died or had another procedure. In angioplasty, a surgeon clears heart arteries using a wire threaded through a vein from the patient's leg. In all the angioplasty patients, the surgeon also implanted a mesh device to keep the arteries open.

Stephen Gielan of the University of Leipzig Heart Center suggests that the exercise therapy benefits the whole cardiovascular system, whereas angioplasty plus the mesh implant open clogged arteries only at particular sites.

Gielan also notes that the no-surgery therapy saved money. Even with the costs of the training in the hospital, "exercise training was associated with about half the costs of the [surgical] intervention," says Stephan Gielan of the University of Leipzig Heart Center.

Because the physicians were worried that exercise- in this case, biking-could strain the patient's hearts, the patients started their training in the hospital. For 2 weeks, they biked six times a day, 10 minutes a session. They then went home and kept up a routine of at least 20 minutes of biking each day.

"The role of physical activity is supported by masses

of data," says Russell V. Luepker of the University of Minnesota at Minneapolis-St. Paul. "The issue is how we get people to do it."

This article was reported in the December 7, 2002, issue of Science Digest.

Making Exercise Easy

While some people may enjoy the group rapport and support of joining a gym, that's not the only way to get your daily exercise. In fact, walking is one of the easiest and least expensive forms of exercise, and as beneficial as any that you will find. If you've avoided physical activity for most of your life, here are a few pointers that will help you make this an easy and enjoyable part of your life.

• Wear comfortable shoes. Without them, your feet will hurt – and you won't stick with it.

• Incorporate a warm up and a cool down session as part of your session. Before you take off at full speed, start with some easy ambling. This allows your heart to build up to a more strenuous pace comfortably.

• Stretch when you are done – your muscles will appreciate it and you will lessen the possibility of soreness the next day.

• Start slowly. When you tell yourself you are going to walk an hour a day, seven days a week, you set yourself up for failure. When you don't do it, you quit. So, tell yourself you are going to do whatever is achievable for you – even if it's just ten minutes or even if it's just parking your car a little further away than usual. Small steps count. Start with a pace where you can walk and talk at the same time. Keep it comfortable.

• Aim for three times a week. Three times is enough to begin to establish the habit and to begin to feel some physical and mental benefits.

• Hike outdoors, if possible. Get outside and enjoy nature if you can. It makes it much easier.

• Be a social walker. Walk with other people – good conversation makes a longer walk go much faster.

• Use music. Put on your headphones. Use upbeat, fast paced music to make the time pass quickly. I also like to listen to books on tape – it lets me feed my mind and exercise my body at the same time.

Whatever form you choose for your program to add physical activity to your life, remember that the key is to make it pleasurable. Don't overdo. The benefits come from sticking with a regular program, which you're more likely to do if its fun. Once you've made physical activity a part of your daily lifestyle, you'll feel so much better about your body and about yourself, that you'll wonder why you didn't start sooner!

– CHAPTER SIX –

Fiber

As the preceding two chapters should have made clear by now, ensuring that you get adequate water and exercise are essential to establishing a program aimed at providing you with a Maximum Quality of Life. It's only common sense that you need to keep your body fit, flexible, and well hydrated. Once you understand the roles they play, it's only common sense to figure out how to add these two components to your lifestyle. It's when we examine the way we *eat* that people often begin to get confused. Why is this?

For one thing, the MIC–through the marketers of food products and pharmaceuticals–has done a great job of confusing the issue of nutrition. Focusing on making top dollar for their products, they have discovered that it's better to emphasize things like taste, convenience, and faddish trends than to educate the public about nutrition. Nowhere has this been more evident than in the first of the nutrients we're going to discuss: fiber.

What is Fiber

Fiber is an easily overlooked, but very important part of everyone's diet. Fiber is found in the cell walls of plants. Its primary function is to provide protection and rigidity, allowing the plant to support its own weight. The

most familiar type of fiber is cellulose, which is the substance that forms the "skeleton" of plants. Cellulose is
non-soluble, meaning that it cannot be dissolved in water.
A variant of cellulose, called hemi cellulose, is less
"woody" in texture and provides the support and protection for the interior cells of plants. This substance *is* water
soluble to some degree. Pectin is a form of fiber found in
the cell walls of fruits. Less recognized are the gums and
lignans, two additional forms of fiber.

When we eat foods made from plants and plant products, we consume their fiber along with all of the other
nutrients contained within the plant cells. Fiber, which is
tough, is not readily digested or absorbed by the body the
way those other nutrients are. Instead, the fiber we consume passes through the gastrointestinal tract more or
less intact, until it is ultimately eliminated.

If we can't digest or otherwise process the fiber we
eat—if it simply passes through our system—why is it so
important? Let's look at what the science tells us.

Fiber Helps Your Heart

The Iowa Women's Health Study, a long-term
research project, involved the participation of 34,492
women and investigated the hypothesis that fiber found in
whole grains might contribute to a reduced risk of
ischemic heart disease (IHD) death, that is sudden death.
The study, published in the August 1998 issue of the
American Journal of Clinical Nutrition, confirmed that an
increase in the consumption of whole grain foods is associated with a significant reduction in the risk of death
from IHD. In fact, just three servings of such foods every

day were enough to reduce the risk of dying from a sudden heart attack by 30 percent. There is no drug on the market that shows such a significant impact on the risk of sudden death by heart attack! The study suggests that it's not just the fiber in whole grain foods that provides this reduced risk. In addition to fiber, these foods also contain antioxidants and other nutrients, which contributed to these impressive findings.

A hospital in Kalamazoo, Michigan, decided to test an educational program developed by Dr. Hans Diehl by enrolling 304 people who had an elevated risk of coronary artery disease. The participants were encouraged to exercise 30 minutes a day and to eat a diet of largely unrefined plant foods high in carbohydrates and fiber; low in fat, animal protein, sugar and salt; and virtually free of cholesterol. In four weeks, the improvements in blood test results, blood pressures, weights, and body mass indexes were highly significant. These fantastic results, according to an article published in the November 1998 issue of the *American Journal of Cardiology,* were accomplished *in just four weeks!* Most drugs *take 2 years* to show this much benefit.

In that same issue, Dr. T. Colin Campbell from Cornell University reported on a very large comparative study he did on the inhabitants of 130 villages in China. Fifty adults in each village were analyzed for a variety of nutritional, viral, hormonal, and toxic chemical factors. Dr. Campbell then compared the findings to the results achieved in the United States. He found heart disease was 16.7 times more common in American men than Chinese men and 5.6 times more common in American women than their Chinese counterparts. He also found that the Chinese villagers had a very low incidence of other diseases. He attributed the difference to greater consumption of green vegetables, a markedly lower consumption of sugar and meat, and a greater emphasis on plant protein in the Chinese diet. In addition, the Chinese villagers had no access to the highly processed foods that form so great a part of the American diet. What is significant in the Chinese diet is that by being so heavily skewed to plant-based foods, it is naturally high in fiber.

A 10-year study in Sweden, reported in the June 1999 issue of the *Journal of the American Medical Association,* involved studying the health of 68,782 nurses who had, at the beginning of the study, no diagnosed angina, myocardial infarction, stroke, cancer, or diabetes. The risk of having a heart attack was 47 percent lower in the group who consumed the most fiber. Looking across the population of women, for every 10-gram/day increase in fiber, the risk was reduced 37 percent. No drug discovered to date can boast of figures like that.

In some cases, findings are derived by a review of an existing body of research work. J. W. Anderson, T. J. Hanna, X. Peng, and R.J. Kryscio from the Division of Biostatistics, VA Medical Center and University of Kentucky, reviewed the scientific literature of the past 20 years. They said, "We have systematically reviewed literature from the past 20 years evaluating an association between dietary fiber and CHD. Foods that are rich in dietary fiber, including fruits, vegetables, legumes and whole grain cereals also tend to be a rich source of vitamins, minerals, phytochemicals, antioxidants, and other micronutrients. Each of these foods may be independently contributing to the cardiovascular protective effects of fiber-rich foods."

Further evidence of the value of a high fiber diet comes from the American Health Foundation of New York, which has explored the causes of cardiovascular diseases and the mechanisms underlying the developments of the disease. The foundation reported in the June 2000 issue of the *Journal of the American College of Nutrition* that fruits, vegetables, and whole grains, with their naturally occurring fiber and antioxidants; along with drinking 2 quarts of water each day has a protective effect against heart disease. It further found that drinking green tea contributes to this protective effect.

Harvard researchers have also gotten onto the pro-fiber bandwagon. The February 1996 issue of the *Journal of the American Medical Association* carried their report on a study that monitored the diets of 43,757 male physicians for six years. For those consuming a total of 30 grams of fiber from all sources, there was a 41 percent decrease in chance of having a heart attack. The chance of *dying from a heart attack* was reduced by 55 percent!

Researchers have long noted that the Mediterranean and Asian diets seem to yield a lower risk of heart disease. Dr. L. H. Kushi from the University of Minnesota researched this issue and reported his findings in the June 1995 issue of the *Journal of Clinical Nutrition*, where he noted that higher rates of consumption of fruits, vegetables, and other high-fiber foods lead to lower rates of heart disease, birth defects, and cataracts.

Finally, Dr. D. S. Gray, associated with the Community Hospital Family Practice Residency in Santa Rosa, California, found that fiber reduces diabetes, constipation, certain types of cancer, and heart disease. He recommends increasing water consumption along with increased fiber consumption.

Reduce Your Chances of Dying From the Disease

Research results keep piling up evidence that fiber is a very heart-friendly element of the diet. For example, researchers at Harvard studied the health habits of 75,521 women in the Boston area for 10 years. They found that whole grain intake reduced the risk of having a coronary by 33 percent. After adjusting for obesity, hormone use, multivitamin or aspirin use, physical fitness, and saturated fat consumption; the women who ate the most fiber still reduced their risk by 25 percent. In other words, leanness, hormones, aspirin, exercise, and saturated fat usage all rolled up together decreased risk of heart disease by only an additional 8 percent. The study did not measure Omega-3 consumption, but their findings still indicate that fiber was a primary controlling factor in the reduction of risk for fatal heart disease.

Overseas, the support for fiber in the diet is equally strong. In the Scotland Heart Healthy Study, reported in the November 1999 issue of the *American Journal of Epidemiology*, scientists discovered that a high fiber diet could decrease the chances of having a heart attack or dying of heart disease by 36 percent. Adding antioxidants to the diet helped reduce the risk even further. Meanwhile, in Oxford, England, a study compared the risk of fatal heart attack for 6,000 vegetarians with that of 5,000 meat eaters. Since meat contains no fiber, the vegetarians clearly had the higher fiber consumption rate of the two groups. After monitoring the participants for 12 years, they found the vegetarian diet cut the chances of dying from any disease, not just from coronary disease, by 50 percent. If a drug company could find a drug that would do this, they could charge a king's ransom for their pills.

In Toronto, Canada, Dr. D. J. Jenkins took healthy volunteers and divided them into three groups. One group ate a high fiber (vegetable, fruit and nuts) diet; one group ate a starch-based diet (cereals and legumes); and one group ate a very low fat diet. In just ten days, the markers for a healthy heart increased significantly for the high fiber group. This means that people who partake of a super healthy, natural food diet can improve their health very quickly. The low fat diet improved their health very little. Meanwhile, back in the United Kingdom, Dr. C. Bolton-Smith of the University of Dundee, Scotland, found that high levels of consumption of fiber, along with vitamins C, E, and A, resulted in a reduction in risk of coronaries by 36 percent.

Dr. James Anderson did a study over a period of 20 years at the Veterans Hospital in Kentucky, and found that whole grains are consistently effective at reducing the risk of heart disease, diabetes and cancer. He recommends that Americans double their dietary fiber intake by increasing their consumption of dried beans, oat products, and certain fruits and vegetables for soluble fiber, and wheat bran for insoluble fiber. Benefits noted include lower serum cholesterol, lower risk of coronary heart disease, reduced blood pressure, enhanced weight control, better glycemic control, reduced risk of certain forms of cancer, and improved gastrointestinal function.

Not a New Issue

Before you start thinking that fiber is some newly discovered panacea for heart health, remember that the first high-profile interest in fiber came in the 1970s. Back then, Drs. H. Trowell and D. Burkitt discovered that diets low in fiber led to heart disease and colon problems, based on their research'in Africa. One concern of their report was that as the African diets became Westernized, the prevalence of heart disease increases.

As a result of these and similar findings in the 1970s, high fiber became an overnight buzzword, and food manufacturers were quick to jump onto the bandwagon. Unfortunately, fiber fell out of fashion, or maybe it would be more accurate to say that it was pushed out—by the MIC, which found its profits on anti-cholesterol drugs eroding rapidly. The MIC was very successful: by the early 1980s you rarely heard about high-fiber foods. Thank goodness that the benefits of fiber are once again being recognized within the community of nutrition specialists.

Making Sense of The Science

Clearly, the available research shows that fiber plays an important role in a heart-healthy nutritional plan. The question is how to put the scientific data into practice. Back in the 1970s, when fiber enjoyed a brief period of faddish popularity, the reason that the MIC was able to so effectively appropriate the fiber fad as a marketing tool for its own highly processed products was because people didn't really know how to incorporate naturally occurring fiber as a natural part of their meals. Instead of making whole grains and fresh fruits and vegetables a part of their diets, people found it easier to look for "high fiber" on the labels of highly processed breads and baked goods.

Those fad years gave us some pretty strange products, including bread "enriched" with wood pulp—otherwise known as sawdust! All that many people learned from the experience was that "high fiber" meant unpleasant taste and texture, so it's no wonder they lost interest after a while. That never had to happen. A diet rich in fiber doesn't require that you eat sawdust sandwiches!

What should you do to increase your fiber intake? Here are a few easy-to-follow suggestions:

- Eat a minimum of three whole grain foods per day, and more for even greater benefits

- Eat more green, red, and yellow vegetables

- Replace some of the animal-protein in your diet with protein derived from plants– like legumes, nuts that grow above the ground, seeds, and whole grains

- Increase your consumption of fruits and vegetables—natural sources of a range of fiber types, from cellulose to pectins and lignans.

A lot of people are discovering that adopting a vegetarian diet has the added benefit of helping to greatly increase their fiber intake almost effortlessly, because when you cut back or eliminate meat from your diet you automatically increase your fiber foods intake. Of course, going vegetarian means you have to pay attention to your protein sources in particular, since animal-based foods are the most efficient source of the whole array of amino acids your body needs. Remember what you learned in Chapter 3: if you ignore the cholesterol terrorists and allow yourself to eat eggs (in moderation, of course), you can go a long way in addressing this problem.

We are not saying that you have to get back to baking your own breads, muffins, and other baked goods from scratch. One great development in recent years has been the rise in popularity of health-conscious bakeries that avoid the pitfalls of the big commercial bakeries. Like my own Natural Ovens Bakery, these newer companies specialize in using fresh, naturally grown ingredients and avoid all the preservatives and other chemical short cuts on which the big corporate food manufacturers rely.

Let's get into specifics, here. If you still need help figuring out how to increase the amount of fiber in your diet, here is a chart that will come in handy.

Category	High Fiber Foods
Vegetables	Baked beans, string beans, broccoli, carrots, celery, kale, leeks, lentils, parsley, spinach, summer squash, watercress, zucchini
Fruits	Apples, blackberries, blueberries, cranberries, currants, dates, figs, lemons, olives, prunes, raisins
Breads, Cereals, and Starchy Vegetables	Whole wheat, rolled oats, fortified and stabilized flax, white beans, kidney beans, pinto beans, brown beans, lima beans, bran cereal, wheat bran, rye bread, corn, graham crackers, farina, egg noodles, whole oats, parsnips, peas, popcorn, brown rice, potatoes, white rice, dark rye flour, spaghetti, winter squash, sweet potatoes, white wheat flour, shredded wheat cereal

Where to Get Fiber in Your Diet

A look at the chart shows how easy it can be to increase your fiber intake with foods that your family can enjoy at every meal and even in their snacks. If you keep lots of wonderful high fiber options available, your whole family will take the loss of less healthy alternatives in stride. By getting them accustomed to reaching for healthier snack alternatives—popcorn instead of greasy potato chips, corn bread instead of gooey, high-sugar packaged cakes, and so on—you're helping your kids develop eating habits that will stay with them for the rest of their lives. At the same time, you're cutting their chances, and yours, of eventually developing heart disease and other serious ailments from 30 to 40 percent or more, while dramatically increasing the overall quality of your lives.

Don't stop with fiber! Remember that we don't want to repeat the mistakes of the cholesterol theorists by settling for a simplistic solution. Increasing your fiber consumption is one element of the larger strategy for healthier eating. Another element, and one that is becoming increasingly recognized by the scientific community as key to good heart health and to good health across the board, is coming up in the next chapter. That's Omega-3, and any heart healthy program needs to include these important fatty acids.

- CHAPTER SEVEN -

Omega-3,
One Very Special Type Of Fat

To understand the importance of the Omega-3 fatty acids, it helps to understand the roles played by fats in general in the human body. Many people don't understand just how many and varied fats are, so when they fall for the cholesterol theory's blanket condemnation of fats and cholesterol they end up cutting out some very important nutrients. By taking the time to understand just how your body uses fats, and how many different kinds of fats are available in the foods you eat, you can improve your ability to make intelligent nutritional choices.

What Kinds of Fat Are There

Let's start by looking at all the different kinds of fat found in the foods we eat. They all share the same basic building blocks: carbon, oxygen, and hydrogen. Some fats carry less hydrogen than others. These are the Omega-6 fats, commonly called polyunsaturates, and can actually hinder your body from making good use of other types of necessary fats. Here's the general rundown of the various categories of fats.

• Monounsaturated fats: Unsaturated fats can be monounsaturated or polyunsaturated. Olive oil or canola oils and avocados are examples of monounsaturated fats (MUFA). These are less

solid than their polyunsaturated counterparts
and remain fluid at room temperature.

• Polyunsaturated fats: Corn or safflower oils
are examples of polyunsaturated fats (PUFA).
These fats are very high in Omega-6 fatty acids.

• Saturated fats: Saturated fats (SFAs) are
dense, solid fats that don't melt at room temperature. Most of the saturated fats in our diets
come from animal products, but coconut fat is
also highly saturated. The chief advantage of
saturated fats is that they do not form free radicals at high temperatures.

• Hydrogenated fats: Some fats are processed
to extend their shelf life so the products can
stay on the store shelf for longer periods of
time. Unfortunately, the hydrogenation process
converts the fats into something very much like
plastic, turning it into something that your body
simply wasn't designed to handle. They are
labeled *trans-fats*, and they are the worst of the
worst fats you can consume. These fats block
the body's use of normal essential fatty acids,
and you should avoid them when at all possible.
The trans-fats are so bad that they were banned
in Europe years ago! Science has shown that
they cause much more heart disease than even
saturated fats.

You Must Have Fat

As you can see, there are many different types of fats in our foods. Some of them are essential for your body to function properly. Every single one of your cells must have a little of the essential fatty acids to keep their outer wall, the cell membrane, flexible enough to permit nutrients to pass in and waste products to pass out. Without the essential fatty acids, the walls of your cells become stiff and inflexible and cannot do their jobs efficiently. These important fats are the Omega-3s, and I recommend that those of you who want to explore the subject of these essential fats in greater depth read *Omega-3 Oils: A Practical Guide*, by Donald Rudin and Clara Felix.

For now, though, it's important to understand how your body makes and uses fats. Your body makes fat from fatty acids or sugar. Some fatty acids are called non-essential acids, and your own body makes them, as it needs them. (Non-essential simply means that they aren't essential to include in your diet because your body creates them naturally.) Other fats, however, cannot be obtained except through the foods you eat. These are called essential fatty acids.

Omega-3 and Omega-6 are essential fatty acids. They produce eicosanoids, which are hormones that regulate a wide variety of body processes. The roles that the Omegas play in producing these hormones is one reason why they are so important for your body's proper functioning, including the way that your body handles cholesterol in the blood. The problem is that, in the United States, people are consuming far too much Omega-6 fatty acids.

The role played by fatty acids in regulating cholesterol in your blood is well documented. In their book,
Omega-3 Oils, Dr. Donald Rudin and Clara Felix provide
this simple explanation:

> Cholesterol doesn't dissolve in water, which
> means it can't move through the bloodstream
> by itself. Therefore, the liver combines each
> cholesterol molecule with a long-chained
> essential fatty acid, and then surrounds it with
> a protein. The resulting package, called a
> lipoprotein, is capable of moving through the
> bloodstream.
>
> *Low-density lipoprotein* (LDL) carries choles-
> terol throughout the body for use by the body's
> cells. If LDL levels in the blood become too
> high, or if the LDLs become rancid, the choles-
> terol tends to stick to the walls of the arteries,
> which causes the arteries to become narrower.
> That's why LDL has been called "bad" choles-
> terol. On the other hand, *high-density lipopro-
> tein* (HDL) has been called "good" cholesterol
> because it removes cholesterol from the blood
> and carries it back to the liver. Only when the
> diet provides enough essential fatty acids to
> link up with cholesterol in the liver can choles-
> terol do its many jobs safely.

If your diet is deficient in one of the essential fatty
acid classes, the Omega-3s, you're heading for heart trouble down the road sooner than you think. An Omega-3
deficiency leads to the inflammation that we talked about
in Chapter 3 when we described the way heart trouble and

plugged arteries begin. It's not a simple case of increasing your Omega-3s in your diet to reverse this effect. You also need to *reduce* your consumption of Omega-6s. Why? Omega-6s actually *block* the beneficial effects of Omega-3s!

The reason that fats in general have gotten a bad reputation is because many people simply are unaware that all fats are not created equal. To these people, all fats are bad. They do not realize in fact, it is a combination of consumption patterns that causes the problem. Scientists have found that when diets are high in cholesterol and Omega-6 fats, they are generally low in alpha-linolenic acid (Omega-3), fiber, and other important nutrients. This *unique combination of excesses and deficiencies* can cause the immune system to malfunction, which leads to heart disease and other chronic degenerative diseases.

Striking the Proper Balance

Polyunsaturated fat (Omega-6) is the fat that cholesterol terrorists have been promoting for curing heart disease for 50 years! This is a real case of preaching false doctrine. This polyunsaturated fat (Omega-6) is what scientists call lino*leic* acid, and is mainly from corn, soybean, safflower and cottonseed oils, and from corn-fed animals. A little Omega-6 is good and you must have it, but a *lot* overexcites the immune system. Omega-3, on the other hand, has the opposite effect of Omega-6 fats; it produces the kind of cellular hormones that *calm* the immune system and are quite anti-inflammatory.

The ratio of Omega-6 to Omega-3 is as important as the absolute amounts of each. In *The Omega Plan*, Dr.

Artemis Simopoulos says that you need to create a ratio of Omega-6 to Omega-3 that is as close to one-to-one as you can get. Most people, who develop out-of-control immune systems and therefore have arthritis, AIDS, heart disease, and other chronic diseases, have an Omega-6 to Omega-3 ratio of *20 to 1 or higher.* The old Eskimo or old Greek societies had a ratio of about 2 to 1. The ratio should never exceed 4 to 1.

In the 1980s, Dr. Donald Rudin and Clara Felix prepared a 'Food Damage Report' that documented changes in the American diet, which have occurred over the past 100 years. Among their findings was a startling discovery that the *consumption of Omega-3s has declined by a full 80 percent!* This change, along with others (including a 50 percent decline in the consumption of B vitamins, a 75 to 80 percent decline in fiber, and a significant loss of trace elements through processing) makes it easy to understand why heart disease is on the rise.

Dr. William Lands, recently retired from the National Institute of Health in Washington, D.C., agrees with Dr. Simopoulos' findings that the 1-to-1, Omega-6 to Omega-3 ratio is best. Dr. Lands has developed a formula that can predict the levels of Omega-3 and -6 in your blood by knowing the Omega-3 and -6 levels in your diet and vice-versa. (See http://ods.od.nih.gov/eicosanoids/index.html and http://ods.od.nih.gov/eicosanoids/KIM_Install.exe for details on analyzing your own diet.) In a case of "better late than never," in September 2002, the National Academy of Science finally got around to putting their stamp of approval on *increasing* Omega-3 in the diet and *limiting* Omega-6!

The National Academy of Science now recommends people already in good health consume 2,000 to 3,000 mg of Omega-3 fatty acids per day (about one tablespoon of ground fortified flaxseed), which is about double the present amount consumed in the average American diet. They also recommend 200 to 800 mg per day of EPA and DHA for protection against coronary heart disease. The NAS stated that levels of 2 to 3 grams per day "afford some protection against coronary heart disease." While they did not address the issue of what people should do who already have heart disease, common sense would dictate that you might need to consume a higher level to correct the problems caused by deficiencies in Omega-3s.

The National Academy of Science also noted that excessive levels of Omega-6s might lead to coronary heart disease and cancer, the two largest killers in America. They recommend an intake level of 10 grams per day and an upper limit of 20 grams per day even though 5 grams a day is enough. For many Americans who have been consuming levels of 30 to 40 grams of polyunsaturated fats in their diet, this is a dramatic reduction. The NAS states that high consumption of Omega-6 fats "creates a pro-oxidant state which may predispose to coronary heart disease and cancer." For the NAS to say that Omega-6 predisposes to heart disease is a *complete about-face* to what they have been strongly saying for the last fifty years. *This welcome reversal in policy is important, because NAS recommendations have a strong influence on the official dietary recommendations put out by the FDA for the benefit of all American consumers.*

Omega-6 fat is truly a case of a highly promoted cure

that makes the disease worse. The "cure" part is that Omega-6 does temporarily lower your serum cholesterol—but then it causes huge inflammation in the arteries. This causes lesions, forcing the body to make extra cholesterol to patch over the lesions. These patches either stay soft and tear loose, which causes sudden blockage of the artery, or they becomes calcified and hard and gradually stop the flow of the blood. The important thing to understand is that all the short-term gains you get from Omega-6 are temporary, and that over time your condition actually *worsens*!

The old-line cholesterol terrorists can't quite understand this process because their theories don't take into account the new information available on the biochemistry of heart disease. Whether they get it or not, the process will kill you and they will get paid. They get away with it because long-standing treatments like theirs, even if they've been disproved by science, are considered legitimate as long as they are deemed "acceptable common practice." In other words, if a treatment or method was used by lots of other physicians in the past, it's okay to keep doing it today, long after that treatment has been demonstrated to be wrong!

The other type of heart disease, arrhythmia (heart beating too fast or too slow) is caused by faulty firing of the automatic pacemaker in the heart. Using tissue cultures of heart cells, Dr. Alex Leaf has very elegantly demonstrated that arrhythmia is caused by a deficiency of Omega-3 in the membranes of the heart. Arrhythmia is a major cause of instant cardiac death, which accounts for about 50% of all deaths from premature heart disease.

This is another reason to *keep Omega-3 levels in the diet as high as possible.*

The Calorie Connection

Another important factor to consider concerning heart disease is excess calories that lead to obvious obesity. Obesity is the "Canary in the Coal Mine" predictor of impending heart disease and diabetes. Dr. K. M. Rexrode from Harvard found that for a man to increase his waistline from 40 to 47 inches, he would increase his risk of heart disease by 60 percent. It didn't make any difference if he increased his waistline with vegetarian fat-free SnackWell's® or T-bone steaks. For females, Dr. Rexrode found that women whose waistlines measured *over 30 inches faced twice the risk of heart disease* as women whose waistlines were under 30.

The excess calories force the body to deal with excess fatty acids in the liver and the bloodstream. This puts a tremendous strain on the immune and inflammatory system, resulting in metabolic disarray. The million-dollar question is, "What drives people to overeat?" This is a hot topic in the medical and scientific world. They can't find an answer because it is right in front of their noses—*overly processed foods.*

People overeat because the food tastes too damn good. Every food company tries to make their foods tastes better and better with artificial flavorings and appetite stimulants so that people will buy more of it. This is a perfectly legal behavior. The additives used are usually nutrient deficient, like sugar, or chemically modified and therefore hard; if not impossible, for the body to metabolize.

We become obese and then develop heart disease or diabetes. You know the rest of the story—premature deaths.

In other words, it doesn't do you any good to switch to "fat-free" food if that substitution means you're boosting your calorie consumption with other non-nutritious foods. Consuming the excess calories means you'll still be facing obesity and probable heart disease down the line, whether the excess calories come from fat or sugar. What is the answer? *Whole foods - high fiber, nutritionally packed foods!* The WE-FOBAM lifestyle and eating plan. Plain and Simple.

The Scientific Community Weighs In

Scientific literature has been full of reports on the harmful effects of too much "polyunsaturated fat" and not enough Omega-3 for many years. One of the earliest reports that Omega-3 is an essential nutrient was published in 1930 by Drs. George and Mildred Burr. In 1965, Dr. Ralph Holman at the University of Minnesota published his findings, which proved that Omega-6 interfered with Omega-3 metabolism. In 1973, Dr. William Lands published his research showing that Omega-6 produces pro-oxidant prostaglandins, which could lead to inflammation and heart disease. More recently, scientists have been exploring the specifics of how the two Omegas really work. Among the important questions this new research has addressed is whether or not the various forms of Omega-3s–which are found in plant foods like flaxseed, walnuts and leafy green vegetables and in fish–are equally beneficial. Here is a small sampling of the research that has been done in recent years.

• In the December 1980 issue of the *American Journal of Clinical Nutrition*, some very astute researchers including Drs. H. O. Bang, J. Dyerberg, and Hugh Sinclair (a personal hero of mine for his pioneering research and steady contributions to the science of nutrition) reported that Eskimos who lived on very high fat/high cholesterol diets had such low rates of heart disease they did not even have a word for it. Eskimos showed no premature deaths from heart disease. The researchers analyzed Eskimos' diets and found they contained lots of Omega-3 fat from eating cold-water fish. The researchers also compared fish eating and non-fish eating cultures and individuals, and found that people who consumed a lot of Omega-3 rich fish had a low risk of dying from heart disease even if they had high blood cholesterol levels.

• Once again in December of 1980, this time in the journal *Prostaglandins*, Dr. W. E. Lands and Dr. B. R. Culp produced the first laboratory evidence that Omega-3 could prevent heart disease.

• The National Heart, Lung, and Blood Institute financed an exciting study, which came out in 2001. This study shows that by increasing Omega-3 intake from a half gram per day to two or more grams per day, the risk of heart trouble was reduced by 40 percent in men and a whopping 58 percent in women. The study found that Omega-3 worked by reducing the inflammatory process, not by reducing cholesterol value. Cutting saturated fat reduced the risk even further. No drug on earth has ever come this close to reducing heart disease by such a factor *and Omega-3 has no bad side effects.*

• Back at the Harvard School of Public Health a major epidemiological study using 43,000 male physicians was conducted, which found that those physicians who consumed at least 2 grams a day of Omega-3 *reduced their risk of a heart attack by 59 percent!* Those who consumed the least saturated fat and cholesterol, compared to those who consumed the most fat and cholesterol, only reduced their risks by 22 percent.

• Finally, there's the 1991 surprise. In 1991, Dr. W. S. Browner was hired by then-Surgeon General, Dr. C. Everett Koop to lead a research team to investigate whether or not eating a high level of saturated fat and cholesterol would dramatically shorten a person's life span. The surprise was that Dr. Browner's team was expected to achieve positive findings–and they did not! Dr. Browner did a scientifically correct, major epidemiological study; but alas, he found that death was hastened by only 3 months in people who ate a high fat diet compared to the government recommended diet of 30 percent fat and not more than 300 mg of cholesterol.

Dr. Koop was livid and tried to prevent the facts from ever being published. The *Journal of the American Medical Association* published the results anyway, giving Dr. Browner the last laugh. Browner even says that the 3-month estimate of delaying death is an overestimate.

Dr. Browner's results shocked many people, but when you think about it you can see why they might be true. Remember, when people cut back on their intake of one kind of food, they're likely to turn to something else to fill the gap. When it comes to fats, people tended to substitute it with foods that contain lots of sugar. The result? Increased obesity and shorter life spans! The low-fat foods of the 90's were nearly all sugar bombs. There's got to be a better way!

The Science Continues

The issue of fats has inspired many prestigious research institutes to establish important epidemiological studies. One, reported in the April 2002 issue of the *Journal of the American Medical Association* by Harvard-based researchers tracked 84,000 nurses over several years. The team discovered that women in the study who consumed fish at least once per week had a 29 percent lower risk of coronary heart disease. The nurses who consumed the most Omega-3s, which are found in many fish, fared even better. They reduced their risk of a coronary by 33 percent!

This research followed on the heels of another major study, published in the same journal in the previous year. That research found that women who ate 5 or more fish meals per week reduced their risk of clot-related death by a full 48 percent. This is much more effective than the results you could achieve by cutting saturated fat or cholesterol consumption in half and taking cholesterol-lowering drugs. It provides you with a much tastier diet, to boot! It isn't only women who reap the benefits, as a 2002 report in the *Journal of Internal Medicine* verifies. In that study, men who reported the highest Omega-3 levels in their blood were a full 80 percent less likely to suffer sudden death from heart disease! Omega-3 is starting to look like a real "wonder drug" in the battle against heart attacks, without ever having to take a pill!

In response to these important results, scientists all over the world are conducting valuable research, leading to a sudden surge in the science available to support the claim that Omega-3s are important. Drs. W. S. Harris and J. H. O'Keefe did a review of the literature published between 1980 and 2000, finding that more than 4,500 reports offering this conclusion had been published between 1980 and 2000. No wonder even the national agencies are finally getting the message!

It's important to remember that heart disease takes many forms. This raises the question of whether the Omega-3s are effective in only some kinds of heart disease. Never fear. Omega-3s have been shown to be important in reducing the risk of arrhythmia, for example, which is when the heart begins to beat extremely slow or extremely fast and refuses to slow down until it becomes exhausted and stops altogether. Dr. Leaf, based at Harvard, offers these conclusions from his research on this issue:

There exists a basic control of cardiac and other excitable tissues by common Omega-3 fatty acids, which has been largely overlooked. With some 250,000 sudden deaths annually largely due to ventricular fibrillation in the US alone, and millions more worldwide, there may be a potential large public health benefit from the practical application of this recent understanding. The knowledge that these fatty acids have direct physical effects on the fundamental property of the nervous system, namely its electrical activity, should encourage further exploration of potential beneficial effects on brain functions both normal and pathological. It seems likely that we are just scratching the surface of the potential health effects of these interesting dietary fatty acids.

Another researcher, Dr. S. C. Renaud, has spent 40 years studying causes of heart disease. Here are his well thought out conclusions, published in the journal *Public Health and Nutrition*:

The Minnesota double-blind intervention trial in psychiatric hospitals has demonstrated that reducing by 50% the intake of saturated fats, replaced mostly by LA, did not lower the rates of nonfatal and fatal MI, even if cholesterol was reduced by 15%. By contrast, three consecutive trials have demonstrated that cardiac death could be lowered by more than 30% without changing serum cholesterol. Among the Omegs-3 fatty acids, ALA appears to be more potent than the longer-chain fatty acids from fish oil in preventing cardiac death. In addition, only ALA lowered nonfatal MI by more than 70%, probably due to direct effect on platelet adhesiveness and aggregation to most agonists, an effect not shared by long-chain Omega-3 fatty acids. Finally, the protection against these main clinical manifestations of CHD developed within weeks, independently of cholesterol.

Dr. Renaud goes on to report in the *Journal of Nutrition, Health and Aging* in 2001, that:

The intake of saturated fat, considered as the main environmental factor for CHD, does not appear to be also closely related to stroke. It has even been observed in the Framingham prospective study, that saturated fats were associated with a protective effect on stroke. The multivariate analysis of the ecological study reported in the present paper suggests that the villain for stroke could be the high intake of linoleic (Omega-6) acid, the main polyunsaturated fatty acid prescribed through the world, to most of the CHD patients. Observation and intervention studies suggest that the fatty acid with the most efficient protective effect on stroke is alpha-linolenic acid (ALA) as for CHD clinical manifestations.

Paul Nestel from the Baker Medical Research Institute, Melbourne, Australia, reports, "vascular function is readily modifiable by nutritional intervention." His work extended beyond the investigation of Omega-3s to include dietary modifications to increase intake of antioxidant vitamins E and C, folate, and isoflavones as well. Regarding the specific role of Omega-3s, he noted "Omega-3 fatty acids derived from fish improved dilation in the microcirculation and also that of larger muscular arteries."

Elsewhere in the world, researchers are continuing to increase our knowledge of the importance of Omega-3s. Dr. C. von Schacky of Germany was moved by the scientific evidence to assert that every physician in the country should begin prescribing Omega-3 for heart disease. The problem is that Omega-3s are not attractive to the MIC because they aren't profitable! *As naturally occurring substances, they can't be patented, so there are no high-priced products to sell.*

That doesn't have to keep you from taking matters into your own hands. You can increase your consumption of fish like tuna and salmon, and use plant foods like stabilized, fortified flaxseed. All these foods are naturally high in Omega-3s, and by making them a regular part of your diet you can realize impressive health results for yourself! For example, you can reduce irregular heartbeats and excessive clotting of the blood–without causing the nasty side effects so often associated with taking drugs. Want more data? Here's a brief world tour of the research:

• The Smart Foods Centre in Australia found that in just 3 weeks on a high flax/soy diet, total cholesterol and LDL cholesterol dropped significantly.

• In Russia, they also found that flaxseed caused "positive dynamic" changes: blood pressure dropped and blood lipids dropped.

• In Germany, researchers found that flaxseed would prevent artery problems and enhance proper prostacyclin formation.

• In Norway, the authorities recommend a diet high in Omega-3 and monounsaturated fat (such as olive oil) and living on a near vegetarian diet. Other Norwegians reported that a diet rich in Omega-3, B-vitamins, fish and plant foods reduced heart attacks, even though blood cholesterol values changed only a small amount.

• In Japan, they found that feeding elderly people 3 grams of Omega-3 per day increased the level of long chain Omega-3 in the blood with no adverse side effects.

• In the Netherlands, amongst people who are at high risk for heart disease even though they are on a high polyunsaturated diet, adding Omega-3 and reducing polyunsaturates decreased high blood pressure and triglycerides.

• In India, where heart disease is rampant in richer areas, Dr. Ghafoorunissa found that increasing the linolenic acid level (Omega-3) and reducing linoleic acid (Omega-6) reduced plugging of the arteries. She recommended regular consumption of plant foods that are good sources of Omega-3.

• An expert workshop in the Netherlands reviewed the health benefits of Omega-3. They recommended that eating fish regularly would reduce heart disease and Omega-3 could alleviate symptoms of arthritis. They made a recommendation that consuming 2 grams per day of Omega-3 would be prudent.

These reports from around the world by many experts prove beyond a shadow of doubt that Omega-3, especially the plant type-linolenic acid, is crucial in the prevention of heart disease and many other chronic diseases. These are not isolated reports from a few individuals. The mechanism of action of Omega-3 has been fully explained. The mechanism of the action of cholesterol is non-existent.

What The Science Tells Us

The lesson to be learned from all this research can be summed up easily. Here are the six points you need to know:

1. Eat Omega-3 rich cold-water fish a minimum of once a week–baked or broiled, <u>not deep fried.</u>

2. Eat a minimum of two grams of Omega-3 per day (one tablespoon of ground flaxseed).

3. Incorporate 1 to 2 tablespoons of ground, fortified flaxseed into your diet every day

4. Reduce polyunsaturates (Omega-6s found in corn, soy, safflower, and cottonseed oil products, among others) as much as possible

5. *Avoid* all excess calories, especially those from saturated fat and sugary foods

6. Eat lots of fruits, and vegetables, and consider taking vitamin C and vitamin E supplements

If you're wondering what kind of quantity to aim for, the answer seems clear. All research seems to suggest that if you include at least two grams of Omega-3 fatty acids in your diet every day, you'll reduce your risk of heart disease dramatically!

Where to Get Omega-3

But how can you reach that goal? The answer is simple–and tasty too! Flax fortified breads, rolls, bagels and cookies are a great source of Omega-3s, as are fish like salmon and sardines. The much maligned egg yolk is another great source, especially if you buy eggs laid by chickens fed on natural grains! Other good choices include raw walnuts, dark green leafy vegetables, and canola and extra virgin olive oils.

Don't expect the MIC to be happy about your choices. We've already mentioned that the MIC is uninterested because there's no potential for profits in pushing Omega-3s. That's why even now many physicians still push the cholesterol test and cholesterol-lowering drugs. Even well intentioned, otherwise highly competent physicians can get brainwashed this way, as I discovered with my own family doctor. After a routine physical about 5 years ago,

I was given the cholesterol test, and my doctor immediately prescribed cholesterol-lowering drugs! Even though he knew my background and training, he simply couldn't shake himself free of the propaganda of the Cholesterol Terrorists long enough to listen to me when I challenged his judgment!

A few weeks later I received dietary guidelines from a dietician, as ordered by my doctor in an effort to "help" me lower my cholesterol. When I saw that they were all focused on cholesterol and mentioned nothing about Omega-3s, even I began to wonder if I ought to be worried about the cholesterol–the terrorists were in my *own* head! So I went back to my own research notes, and thank goodness that I did; otherwise, I might not have noticed that cholesterol-lowering drugs have to be monitored with regular tests for reduced liver function! Great–cut my cholesterol, but destroy my liver!

Like many medical professionals, my physician was simply doing what he had been told to do based on years of MIC propaganda. He saw a number come up on the cholesterol test and that's all he needed to know! He did not check to discover that my Omega-3 status was similar to traditional Japanese and Eskimos who do not die from "heart disease." Even though I told him this, he seemed incapable of understanding why this would matter. He could not deviate from the Cholesterol Terrorists' party line, even when confronted with clinical data!

To be fair, my doctor was a victim of a medical training tradition that treats nutrition education as unimportant. His entire education on the subject was wrapped up in a lecture that lasted just a few hours. With that kind of training, how could he know the dynamics of the Omega-3/Omega-6 balance? He didn't even know that there's a new predictive test for heart disease risk, called the Omega-3 Test™.

Testing for Omega-3

Dr. Doug Bibus and Dr. Ralph T. Holman (inventor of the Omega-3 terminology) have pioneered nutritional assessment based on the fatty acid health assessment and the Omega-3 Test™. This relatively simple, yet sensitive test is predictive of cardiovascular risk by modeling. The Omega-3 Test™ directly measures the amount of Omega-3 and Omega-6 fatty acids in your blood in a special lipid pool called phospholipids which were demonstrated to relate diet and tissue composition of Omega-3 and Omega-6 fatty acids. Drs. Bibus and Holman have literally analyzed thousands of samples of subjects from around the world, including both healthy and diseased populations, to better understand the role of Omega-3 fatty acids in health and disease. Some key findings of this research are that different populations have differing Omega-3 status. Americans are on the bottom of this international list for their Omega-3 status, and diseased Americans have even lower Omega-3 levels. Unfortunately, *one of the lowest populations* reported by Drs. Bibus and Holman were *American infants!*

Omega-3 testing is just catching on and should soon replace cholesterol testing as the "Heart Healthy Test." If you want your blood tested with the Omega-3 Test™ you can contact Dr. Doug Bibus at Lipid Technologies, LLC under www.omega3test.com or write him at PO Box 216, Austin, MN 55912.

The Omega-3 Test™ measures all the different types of fatty acids in the blood and how much there are of each of them. The fatty acids in your blood represent the fatty acids in your diet, much like the old adage that says "You are what you eat!" If you are eating an Omega-3 deficient diet with lots of Omega-6 (like 90 percent of all Americans) your blood will be high in Omega-6 fatty acids like linoleic and arachidonic (AA) acids and low (deficient) in good fat, Omega-3 fatty acids like alpha-linolenic acid, eicosapentaenoic acid (EPA) and docosahexaenoic acid (DHA). Additionally, the ratio between the Omega-6 fatty acids (that produce the highly inflammatory eicosanoids) and Omega-3 fatty acids (that battle the inflammatory response) is used as a marker of inflammatory potential or how excited your immune system gets when it is "turned on." Remember that too much of the inflammatory response or a hyperactive immune response is now reported to be a major cause in the development of heart disease.

Getting tested can tell you if you are one of the millions of Americans who are deficient in Omega-3 fatty acids. It can also tell you if you are at risk for heart disease and will help you find a diet or supplemental regimen that can help you improve levels of Omega-3 in your blood, body and immune cells.

Work by Holman and Bibus has not only highlighted the significance of Omega-3 in the diet, but also has reported some of the potential consequences of not having enough. Nutritional assessment of several international populations has highlighted how deficient Americans are in Omega-3 (Table 6-1).

Population	Percent of Fatty Acids in Blood		
	Total Omega-3	Total Omega-6	Ratio (ω6/ω3)
Nigerians	13.4	30/3	2.26
Northern Swedes	13.1	35.8	2.73
Keralites (India)	10.4	29.2	2.8
Southern Swedes	8.68	37.4	4.31
Australians	7.35	39.9	5.43
Minnesota Omnivores	5.53	42.6	7.70
Minnesota Vegetarians	5.48	42.1	7.68
Bulgarians	5.26	41.0	7.79

From this data, it is clear that populations consuming fish like the Swedes and Kerala Indians have good Omega-3 status. Populations like the Nigerians, who consume some fish but also considerable amounts of grains and vegetables and very little vegetable oil or processed foods, also have excellent Omega-3 status. Thus the strategy to good Omega-3 status is to reduce your Omega-6 intake and increase your Omega-3 intake.

Figure 6-1 also represents the competitive nature of Omega-3 and Omega-6 fatty acids for assimilation into blood and tissue. People with high levels of Omega-6 (most Americans) have low levels of Omega-3. People with high levels of Omega-3 have low levels of Omega-6. This balancing act in the blood between Omega-6 and Omega-3 is the key to your health. You need healthy amounts of Omega-3 circulating in your blood and balance between Omega-6 and Omega-3 fatty acids in your body so that your immune response is balanced. Remember that a hyperactive immune response is a major cause of heart disease and balance between Omega-6 and Omega-3 in the blood is key to keeping heart disease from developing.

The conclusion to the Omega-3 and Omega-6 discussion is finally complete. The national governing body on recommended intakes for all U.S. citizens has finally put their official "Stamp of Approval" on increasing Omega-3 in the diet to at least 2000 to 3000 mg per day and limiting Omega-6 to 10 to 20 grams per day.

Omega-3 has now attained the high status of a nutrient that can really make a significant difference! It is *a nutrient that has been conclusively shown to reduce deaths not only from heart disease but also cancer,* the two biggest killers in America.   In the last 50 years, Omega-6 (polyunsaturates) has gone from being an agent considered effective in the prevention of heart disease (because it lowered cholesterol) to an agent that will actually *cause* heart disease — *because it causes excess oxidation.* The Omegas aren't the whole story. Let's move on to look at another important aspect of the WE-FOBAM program: the very important B-vitamins, essential in any heart-healthy lifestyle.

CHAPTER EIGHT

B-Vitamins And Folic Acid

Two of the B vitamins—B6 and B12—along with folic acid are very important in keeping you heart-healthy. They work by removing toxins formed when your body breaks down animal protein during metabolism. These toxins, in particular a toxic amino acid metabolite from methionine called homocysteine, can cause serious health problems. Even if you currently suffer from a high level of homocysteine in your system, an adequate B-vitamin intake can work wonders in detoxifying and eliminating it as a health threat!

Folic acid is important for another reason as well, thanks to the research results that began to be published during the 1980s. That's when scientific circles began to recognize the importance of folic acid for pregnant women because of its role in preventing birth defects. Even so, it took more than a decade before the Food and Drug Administration took the hint. The FDA now requires grain millers to add small amounts of folate (folic acid) to their products, but that policy was only put into effect in the year 2000! The good news is that the FDA got around to doing it at all: shortly after the policy's institution, birth defects in the United States dropped significantly. The bad news is that it took the FDA so long. Think of all the children born with birth defects that might have been prevented if only the FDA had acted more quickly. I wonder how many other types of birth defects could be prevented by good nutrition.

Don't make the mistake of thinking that folic acid only matters during pregnancy. Folate and all the B vitamins are important for every organ of your body—especially your heart! So let's take a look at the science that backs this up.

The B Vitamin Group

Scientists today are excited about folate, also commonly known as folic acid, but this is only one of several important nutrients in the group known as the B vitamins. Other important B vitamins include B-1, also called thiamin; B-2, also called riboflavin; B-3, also known as niacin; B-6, also called pyridoxine; and B-12, also called cobalamin. Each plays a significant role in keeping your body functioning properly and all of them are important in maintaining good heart health, but when it comes to preventing heart disease and returning a damaged cardiovascular system to better health, the three to keep in mind are B-6, B-12, and folic acid.

The problem is that the B vitamin complex is one of the most neglected classes of nutrients in most Americans' diets. This is especially important because B-6 and folic acid are not stored in your body, so you need to include them in your meals *every day*. B-12, on the other hand, is stored in the liver.

So what do these important nutrients do for you? Let's start with B-12, which helps your body maintain healthy nerve and red blood cells. Because your body stores it, you don't need to get a specific amount of B-12 into your diet every single day—it's enough that you make sure you're getting a regular supply. Still, since it is so important to your health, why not make the effort? It's found in meat, fish, and poultry, as well as in eggs and fortified breads. Deficiencies in B-12 show up in symptoms like weakness, fatigue, constipation, and flatulence. Even more troubling is when a B-12 deficiency leads to neurological damage, which results in symptoms like a tingling in the hands and feet, depression, confusion, and memory loss.

Fortunately for many of us meat eaters, the abundance of B-12 in animal products makes it unlikely that we will suffer a B-12 deficiency unless we suffer from certain kinds of anemia or other disorder that inhibit the absorption of this nutrient, which often happens upon aging. Even modified vegetarian diets, if they include eggs, provide the B-12 you need. Strict vegetarians need to take care to ensure that they are getting B-12 if they totally avoid animal-based foods. Fortified grain products are–for this group–the best way to go, and supplements are another good idea.

Vitamin B-6 is a water-soluble, non-stored vitamin that helps your body metabolize Omega-3 and other fats and build new body tissues. Because of its fat-metabolizing function, the amount of B-6 you need is directly related to the amount of animal foods–with their high fat content–in your diet. B-6 is found in a wide range of foods, from fruits and vegetables to animal products and grains. Unfortunately, even though it is present in our foods, most Americans don't get enough of this vitamin. One reason is because it is water-soluble, which means that it can be lost during cooking if much water is used in the process. That's why your best bet is eat your foods cooked in little water, and when it comes to vegetables and fruit, raw is the best choice of all.

Finally there's folic acid, which has excited a lot of interest because of its recently discovered role in preventing certain kinds of birth defects, but which is also of significant benefit to your heart's health. Folic acid occurs in a wide range of plant-derived foods–from berries to legumes and whole grains, and from citrus fruits to dark, leafy green vegetables. Again, it is a water-soluble nutrient, so it is best to eat these foods raw or cooked in as little water as possible and for only a short time.

While it is always best to get as much of your body's nutrients in natural form as possible, the B vitamin complex is so important that you may want to consider supplements as well. In fact, now that the FDA has finally gotten with the program–at least with regard to folic acid, the agency has ordered that many products be enriched to enhance their B vitamin content, and it recommends that people, especially pregnant women, take folic acid in supplement form.

The Scientific Data on the B-Complex

There has been a flurry of excitement in vitamin B research since the late 1980s, although those who work in the field of nutrition knew about them for many decades. What's most exciting is that the research indicates more than a preventive role for these nutrients. In other words, research indicates that B vitamins can actually reverse damage that has already occurred, in part because of how well they work in reducing already high homocysteine levels. Here are a few important findings of recent science:

- Epidemiologists at the Harvard School of Public health conducted a survey and found that people who consumed twice the recommended daily allowance (RDA) of folate had 31 percent less heart trouble, *even if they were already on a low fat, high fiber diet.* Their findings, published in the February 1998 issue of the *Journal of the American Medical Association,* also indicated that people who consumed 3 times the RDA for B-6, along with twice the RDA of folate, had 45 percent less risk of heart disease.   These dramatic findings are particularly important when you compare the results to those achieved by any of the standard drug treatments currently used to combat heart disease. Unlike drugs, B-6 and folate have *no* negative side effects, many *positive* side effects, and they cost only pennies per day.

- Dr. D. S. Wald of the Department of Cardiology in Sussex, England, was also interested in the role of folic acid for achieving and maintaining heart health. He studied 151 patients who already suffered from ischemic heart disease, hoping to learn how much of this nutrient was needed to begin to repair the damage. He found that a minimum of .8 milligrams per day was needed to achieve the healing effect desired, and notes that this is twice the level recommended by the United States nutrition guidelines. That means you can't go by the FDA's recommendations, and that the FDA standards for enriching foods with B-complex vitamins, while they might help in the fight against birth defects, won't make any impact on reversing the damage of ischemic heart disease.

• In the January 2001 issue of *Clinical Cardiology*, Dr. A. U. Chai at the University of New Mexico Health Center affirmed that elevated homocysteine levels are now viewed as a risk factor for coronary artery disease, and that folate supplementation was a safe and effective way to prevent heart disease. While calling for more research to develop his findings further, he recommends a minimum of 400 micrograms of folate daily, whether consumed in the normal diet or achieved through supplementation.

• Dr. S. R. Maxwell from the Department of Medicine at the University of Edinburgh has been reporting for the last 30 years that folate deficiency leads to damage of the arteries, especially when antioxidant levels were also low. He is no doubt gratified that the rest of the world seems to be catching up to him, but he cautions against taking an overly simplistic approach to the problem. He stresses that we need to look at both our folate levels *and* our antioxidant consumption. Adding only antioxidants to a ravaged system at that point does not do much good as the folate and other nutrients are also necessary for healing.

• Let's not forget the French. Dr. C. M. Tribouilloy at the University of Picardie, reporting in the December 2000 issue of *Chest*, found that the greater the deficiency of folate, the greater the possibility that an individual will develop atherosclerosis and that the damage to the arteries increases substantially as the folate deficiency worsens.

• Meanwhile, back in the United States, Dr. P. O. Kwiterovich Jr. from the John Hopkins University Lipid Clinic, and Department of Pediatrics, John Hopkins University Medical School, Baltimore, Maryland, led a study that looked into other B vitamins, particularly niacin. His work, reported in the November 1998 issue of the *American Journal of Cardiology*, demonstrated that niacin can increase HDL particles far more than any drug and can reduce the risk of heart disease. Niacin is a common treatment recommended by the more nutritionally enlightened physicians, but it cannot get the job done alone. Instead, it should be made a part of the broader lifestyle we call the WE-FOBAM lifestyle.

Why Wait For the FDA

Given the speed with which the government moves, it will take many more years for the FDA to officially raise the RDA to **optimum** levels. While we wait for our government to get around to listening to what the scientists have been telling us for more than a decade, we are losing people needlessly to heart disease. Some estimates about the economic impact of the simple enhancement of our B vitamin consumption suggest that we could see a $20,000 *decrease* in the cost to treat heart disease compared to conventional treatment for *each life-year saved*. Maybe that's the problem! This kind of savings is good news for you, your friends, and me, but not so good for the drug and surgery industries.

The savings from an enlightened approach to B vitamins can really mount up. Researchers at the University of California looked into the question and estimate that prescribing a B-vitamin supplement to all people with symptoms of heart disease would save $2 billion dollars over ten years and dramatically improve the quality of life for heart disease suffers. That would take a big bite out of the MIC's revenues, to be sure, so don't expect the Cholesterol Terrorists to start advocating this kind of treatment any time soon. In fact, the MIC has a history of going to the opposite extreme. Through its powerful lobbies, it managed to get the FDA to suppress recommendations on folic acid and other non-drug, heart-healthy nutrients for years. It was only in 2000, when a federal court stepped in, that the FDA retreated from this obstructionist position and stepped out of the way.

Today, in the few short years since the FDA "gag order" against publicizing the smart-nutrition approach to heart health, we're suddenly seeing news popping up all over the place, telling us how we can better protect our hearts and arteries with nutritional strategies like increasing our B-vitamin consumption. The timing is no coincidence. The research has been with us for decades, but the ability to spread the word was lacking. Now that it's permissible to get the news out, researchers are making up for lost time—and hoping to avoid any more needless lost lives.

Taking Charge of Your Health

The message of the researchers working with the B vitamins is clear. We all need to consume more than the RDA of folate, and it's a good idea to take a balanced vitamin supplement as well. The shame is that, as a nation, most of us are deficient to some degree in these very important nutrients even though they are readily available in a wide variety of tasty, healthful foods. You don't have to look very hard to find great sources of folate, for example, now that the FDA has ordered that many baked goods be enhanced. You can add to that source simply by making sure that you also include legumes, wheat germ, nuts, seeds, eggs, fish, and a whole host of other great, fresh foods to your diet. We really can wipe out B vitamin deficiencies in our lifetime, and enjoy some great tasting foods while we're at it!

CHAPTER NINE

Antioxidants

Everybody knows that you can't live without oxygen. Without it, our bodies cannot extract the energy they need from the food we eat. It is so important to our survival that we cannot last more than a few minutes without taking another breath of it. While it is vitally necessary to our continued life and health, it also produces damaging byproducts when it is used in normal metabolic processes. These byproducts, called free radicals, are chemical compounds that increase the probability that we will develop any of a wide range of infections and degenerative diseases, including cancer, diabetes, heart attacks, premature aging, and strokes. Free radicals do this by causing cellular damage—not unlike the way oxygen causes unprotected iron to rust (rust is the result of oxidation in metal). This cell damage weakens the immune system and is a factor in heart disease and in speeding up the aging process.

To avoid the damage that free radicals can do, a healthy approach to nutrition must include substances that will protect the body's cells from free radicals. These substances are called antioxidants, and among the better known are vitamin C, vitamin E, and beta-carotene. Antioxidants do their work in any one of several different ways. Here's a list of the variety of methods by which antioxidants help keep your body healthy.

- Control the production of free radicals

- Transform free radicals into less harmful substances

- Repair the cell membranes and chromosomes that have already suffered free-radical damage.

While everybody has probably heard of the "big three" antioxidants–vitamin C, vitamin E and beta-carotene, there are some other nutrients that also get the job done. Among the less well known of these nutrients are the polyphenols, also known as catechins, proanthocyanidins, isoflavones and flavonoids. Like their better-known antioxidants, these substances can dramatically improve and extend your life and reduce your chances of dying from heart disease and other chronic disorders. Recent research has increasingly focused on how these nutrients contribute to your total heart health.

Polyphenols and Heart Disease

Polyphenols are a special group of antioxidants found in fruits, vegetables and whole grains. There are about 4,000 different polyphenols found in foods. Not one of them is 'essential' but as a group they are very important and contribute more antioxidant power to the diet than vitamins C, E, and beta-carotene combined. Some of the especially rich sources of polyphenols include blueberries, cranberries, apples, onions, green tea, red wine, PAC sorghum, and whole-wheat bran.

Outside of the human body, this large group of antioxidants is what gives fruits and vegetables their bright colors. Some are soluble in water, while others are insoluble, and this is an important distinction for those of us who want to maximize our heart health. This is because the polyphenols that are insoluble may act as antioxidants in the intestinal tract by preventing the formation of toxic compounds, while the water-soluble ones are absorbed into the bloodstream and prevent toxins from forming in all parts of the body.

Remember, though, that polyphenols are a widely varied group of nutrients, and not all of them are found in every general polyphenol source. For instance, grapes contain the polyphenol groups called resveratrol and anthocyanidins, whereas teas and sorghum contain a group called catechins. Onions and apples, on the other hand, contain quercetin. A special kind of sorghum, known as PAC sorghum, is extremely rich in the polyphenols known as proanthocyanidins. Research is underway that suggests that PAC sorghum acts as a booster, increasing your body's antioxidant power and reducing oxidative stress.

What Does The Science Say

Let's get right into the specific research on antioxidants, which first began to truly excite scientists more than two decades ago. For example, in the years from 1981 to 1984, researchers at Tufts University, in Boston, Massachusetts, conducted a study of 725 healthy college seniors in an effort to assess their dietary habits, particularly noting their intake of vitamin C. Ten years later they returned to their study participants, this time to assess their health status. The results were clear: those students who initially reported a diet high in vitamin C showed a 45 percent improvement over their fellow participants when it came to risk of death from diseases of all kinds, and a whopping 62 percent reduction when it came to the risk of death from heart disease. The importance of vitamins, and vitamin C in particular, seemed clearly linked to a reduction in the risk of heart disease. Best of all, there are no negative side effects to a diet rich in the fruits and vegetables from which we get this important vitamin.

A team led by Dr. L. H. Kushi of the University of Minnesota, who in early 1986 circulated a questionnaire to 34,486 postmenopausal women of good health, enquiring about their dietary habits with particular emphasis on their vitamin intake. The team then followed these women for seven years to see if there were any implications for heart health. The results, reported in 1996 in the *New England Journal of Medicine* were particularly significant with regard to vitamin E—from foods, not from supplements. The women who consumed the most vitamin E from their normal foods had a 58 percent less chance of dying from heart disease, even if their consumption of other vitamins was low!

Dr. D. K. Pandey and his associates at the University of Texas carried out an even longer-term study, spanning 40 years. Their interest was in vitamin C and beta-carotene, and they tracked 1,556 middle-aged men employed by Western Electric, a firm located in Chicago, Illinois. Comparing vitamin intake with incidence of heart disease and death, they discovered that those employees who consumed the most vitamin C and beta-carotene in their normal foods cut their risk of dying from heart disease by 30 percent. The health benefits didn't stop there!

The risk of dying from cancer was cut by 40 percent, and the risk of dying from any other cause was also cut by 30 percent. Drugs don't have such multiple benefits and without any side effects.

These impressive results have been reproduced and confirmed by research done around the world. In Japan, for example, Dr. T. Yokoyama followed the diet of 2,000 men and women for 20 years. The group receiving the most vitamin C **from their food** had 41 percent less chance of having a stroke. A shorter-term study conducted in the Netherlands had researchers following 4,800 elderly subjects for 4 years, tracking the effects of beta-carotene in the diet. They found those receiving the most beta-carotene **from food** had a 45 percent less chance of developing heart disease. In Finland, Dr. K. Nyyssonen took on the problem from a different direction. Nyyssonen followed the diet of 1,600 men for 8 years, taking special note of those whose diets were *deficient* in vitamin C. He found those who were most deficient in vitamin C had 3.5 times greater chance of having a heart attack. After adjusting for fiber intake, carotene intake, and saturated fat intake, the deficient men had 2.5 times the risk. Finally, back in the United States, Dr. W. S. Browner from the Veteran Affairs Medical Center in San Francisco found a 27 percent decrease in the prevalence of heart disease among veterans who consumed the most vitamin C compared to those who consumed the least. Vitamin C worked much better at reducing the risk of heart disease than lowering overall fat content in the diet.

Research into the polyphenols has had equally encouraging results. Here's a whirlwind tour of some of the findings:

- On the subject of polyphenols, the latest research is very encouraging. In 1997, researchers at the National Public Health Institute in Finland reported on their study of 25,000 randomly selected men, which demonstrated the effectiveness of 18 mg polyphenols per day. At this level, the subjects showed a 23 percent reduction in the incidence of instant-death heart attacks, even among smokers, when compared to the results for participants whose intake was 4 mg per day.

- The same study looked at the effect of polyphenol consumption in women, where they found that those who consumed the most polyphenols reduced the risk of dying from a heart attack by 46 percent. The polyphenol source for both study populations was primarily apples and onions. These are easy-to-serve, everyday foods.

- Meanwhile, Harvard researchers did a study of the diets of 34,000 male physicians and came up with similar findings. They found that those who consumed the most polyphenols reduced their chance of dying from a heart attack by 37 percent, compared to those who consumed the least polyphenols.

- In another long-term study of 805 older men

by Drs. M. G. Hertog and D. Kromhout, the intake of several specific polyphenols was measured. The major sources were green tea, onions, and apples. The group who consumed the most polyphenols reduced their risk of heart disease by 58 percent. After adjusting for smoking, cholesterol intake, obesity, blood pressure, exercise, coffee, vitamins C and E, the risk reduction was even greater – 68 percent.

• Dr. J. H. Weisburger from the American Health Foundation in New York reviewed the scientific literature on polyphenols, hoping to discover the most effective consumption levels for the prevention of disease. He concluded that Americans need to consume 5 to 9 servings a day of fruits and vegetables in order to obtain adequate levels of polyphenols to protect themselves from heart disease and some cancers.

• Drs. D. K. Das and A. Bertelli had a different research interest. They wanted to explain the 'French Paradox' (high fat diet; low incidence of heart disease in France) by noting that the high level of certain compounds in red wine protected people from heart disease, even when they were extracted from the red wines and given as a pill. This demonstrates that it is not the 'atmosphere' of relaxing and having a glass of red wine that protects the French people, but it is actually a group of polyphenols found in red wine. Aw, shucks. It just can't be the diet, can it?

• A second study by Dr. I. C. Arts from the Netherlands found that high levels of catechins (a type of polyphenol) reduced the chances of having an instant death heart attack by 51 percent in elderly men. Catechins did not significantly reduce the chances of having coronary thrombosis.

• Drs. P. C. Hollman and M. B. Katan, again reporting from the Netherlands, found that the natural polyphenol present in onions was absorbed twice as well as the purified, isolated compound. This shows the advantage of food over pills.

• Drs. F. Visioli and C. Galli, of the University of Milan, in Italy, found that virgin olive oil contained potent polyphenols which were exceptionally good scavengers of free radicals that harm the lining in the walls of the arteries and start the process called 'heart disease.' They found the greener the virgin olive oil, the more protection.

• Again from Italy, Dr. M. Serafini conducted a study that showed even alcohol-free red wines dramatically reduced harmful oxidative products from forming in the blood stream within one hour of consumption. So even those who prefer to avoid drinking alcohol can benefit from the antioxidant effects of red wine!

• Drs. R. A. Jacob and B. J. Burri from the USDA Agricultural Research Center in San

Francisco reviewed the scientific literature and found that the data, "suggests that protection against oxidative damage and related disease is best served by the variety of antioxidant substances found in fruits and vegetables."

• Drs. A. J. Baublis and E. A. Decker from the Coca Cola Company in Atlanta, Georgia, report that whole wheat and wheat bran are important sources of dietary antioxidants. They found the polyphenolic acids from a single serving of whole-wheat possessed strong antioxidant activity. (Coming to a store near you – whole-wheat Coca Cola.)

• Last, but certainly not least, Dr. Dean Kromhout from the Division of Public Health Research, National Institute of Public Health and the Environment, Bilthoven, The Netherlands, reported that the Seven Countries Study showed the level of oxidized fat increased mortality and the level of polyphenol flavonoids reduced the long-term death rate from oxidized fat.

By this time, you should certainly be getting the picture.

Putting The Science to Practical Use

There you have it. Studies from respected institutions in Texas, Minnesota, Boston, Finland, Japan and Italy all say the same thing: A diet high in antioxidants can have a profound effect on your heart health and longevity. In other words, it really pays to eat fortified foods, fruits, and vegetables. The benefits of the fruits and vegetables were far higher than one would expect based on just the known vitamin content. So now it is up to us, as consumers, to put that science to practical use in our daily lives—to develop a nutritional plan of action that significantly boosts our bodies' supply of these important substances.

What Would Such a Plan of Action Include

First, you want to look at your daily food intake. Are you getting a good variety of vegetables and fruit every day? Make sure you're regularly consuming apples and onions. When reaching for a beverage, green tea, purple grape juice, and red wine are all great sources of antioxidants, too—and for the teetotalers among us, alcohol-free red wine is just as good an antioxidant source as its alcohol-bearing cousin. To improve your intake of carotene, make sure your diet includes carrots, sweet potatoes, and squash—every day.

How much is enough? For vitamin C, the science indicates that 2,000 mg is a good daily goal. For vitamin E, many studies suggest that you should aim for about 200 mg daily. For the polyphenols, much of the research indicates that you should be aiming for at least 300 mg daily. The question is, "How do you achieve these dietary goals?" Make sure you get lots of fresh fruits and vegetables at every meal. To make it easier, here's a list of rich sources of the various antioxidants:

Phytoestrogens –

• Fruits: Purple grapes, apples, cranberries, strawberries

• Vegetables: soybeans, legumes, onions, broccoli

• Beverages: Soy milk, red wine, purple grape juice, dark beer

• Other sources: cereals and dark chocolate

Beta-carotene –

• Red, yellow and orange fruits and vegetables,

• Dark green leafy vegetables like kale, romaine, beet greens, broccoli, carrots, tomatoes, peaches, cantaloupe

Vitamin C –

• Citrus fruits and juices (including melons, strawberries, papaya, kiwis, raspberries) and cruciferous vegetables (broccoli, cauliflower, Brussels sprouts, and cabbage)

Vitamin E –

• Vegetable oils, whole grains, fortified cereals, nuts, dark leafy greens, wheat germ

Polyphenols –

• Onions, apples, PAC sorghum, green tea, red grapes, blueberries

There you have it. A diet rich in whole grains, vegetables, fruits, and nuts is clearly your best choice—and a quick review of the foods listed above shows how delicious an antioxidant-rich diet can be.

CHAPTER TEN

Minerals

We are finally coming to the end of the WE-FOBAM program of nutrition and exercise. The final item on the list, minerals, is by no means last in importance. Minerals play a vital role in every metabolic step in the human body. They help to break down food into its individual building blocks, and then they help put these building blocks back together to make up the various parts of our body. Without minerals our body would not function at all, and we would lack such basic items as our bones, and our finger and toenails.

Learning to design a nutritional program that guarantees appropriate consumption of minerals can be tricky, because minerals are powerful compounds. Too much is just as dangerous as not enough. Each mineral is just as important as all the others, so getting a lot of one just won't make up for lack of another one. In fact, an excess of one can interfere with the absorption and metabolism of another mineral.

Having said that all minerals are important, the WE-FOBAM program pays special attention to what we think of as the "Big Nine." This is not because you can do without the rest, but because the American diet is particularly likely to be deficient in these. This is true even for the best known of the bunch, calcium!

Calcium

Calcium gets a lot of attention in the media, particularly in reports on women's health issues, because of its supposed role in maintaining strong bones for post-menopausal women who face an increased risk of osteoporosis. In fact, the prevalence of news about calcium leads many people to think that it is the *only* mineral that is important. Nothing could be further from the truth. Even worse, as a result of this excess promotion some people consume too much calcium, thinking that if a little is good, lots more would be better. This is a very bad idea, because an excess amount of calcium actually interferes with the absorption of other necessary minerals. The trouble doesn't stop there. Some of the more popular sources of calcium also come with excess phosphate, a lot of extra calories, and appetite enhancers, all of which can really pack on the pounds. All this frenzy over calcium may even be misplaced! No five-year (or longer) studies of high milk diets have been done to show that they can actually prevent osteoporosis, arthritis or joint degeneration. As a matter of fact, researchers from Harvard have shown that increased hip and forearm fractures are associated with increased milk consumption.

Your body does require calcium, so you do want to make sure that you're getting some in your diet. Many people, particularly older women, opt for calcium supplements, "just to be on the safe side." Keep in mind that calcium supplements alone won't do you any good if it isn't accompanied by adequate levels of vitamin D: without that vitamin, your body won't absorb the calcium, so you're getting no benefit from it at all. According to many studies, American's consume far too little vitamin D. Our principle source of that vitamin isn't even in our foods—it comes from exposure to sunlight! As our society turns away from a lifestyle oriented to outdoor activities, we're getting precious little exposure to the sun. As a result, many high-calcium products like milk and cheese are often fortified with vitamin D. Another good and more natural source is the egg—egg yolks are one of the few good natural sources of the vitamin.

Calcium has its downside, too. This mineral is usually found in combination with phosphate in the diet of soda pop lovers, and together they form a significant factor in increasing blood pressure and hardening of the arteries. With all the pressure put on women to increase milk consumption, it is no wonder their rates of heart disease are skyrocketing. Many authorities have come to feel that excess calcium and phosphate are major contributors to the rising death toll from heart disease. Calcium in cows' milk presents its own peculiar problems. While it is the perfect food for a baby calf, it contains high levels of protein, and the acid ash that is burned off from the metabolism of that protein can actually leach the structural calcium of your bones! Remember, *even baby calves stop drinking cows' milk after only a few months of life!* For the rest of their lives they depend on the *vegetation* they graze to get needed calcium.

Of course, I'm not advocating that you cut calcium from your diet. I just want you to understand that calcium is a two-edged sword: you need to be very careful about how much of it you consume. Even if your biggest concern is the prevention of osteoporosis, you must remember that this is a complex condition and just increasing your calcium intake can't solve it. In fact, Dr. S. Seely, writing in the November 1991 issue of the *International Journal of Cardiology*, states that the average worldwide calcium requirement for young adults is only 300 to 400 mg per day, which is a lot less than what the dairy dominated Nutritional Research Council promotes.

From a world-wide perspective, we know that scientific bodies in most countries in the world recommend on average 400 mg per day, but in countries with large dairy lobbyists, the RDA level is set much higher. Dr. Seely argues that the hazard of a high intake results in calcium being deposited inside the arteries to act as cement, making the plaque harder as it calcifies the saturated fat and foam cells. Calcium also makes the walls of the arteries more rigid. This makes the heart work harder in two ways: the artery walls are less elastic and the arteries are more plugged. There are multiple ways to solve this problem – either consume less calcium, consume more phytic acid from whole grains, consume more magnesium to balance out the calcium, or take a calcium antagonist drug. You already know my opinion of throwing money at the pharmaceutical arm of the MIC, but Dr. Seely's findings bear me out. He says that the calcium antagonist is the *least* desirable alternative.

Calcium from a diet consisting largely of fruits, vegetables, and whole grains is highly available, if the diet is moderate in protein, fat, and salt. This is why people on the WE-FOBAM diet do not need a calcium supplement, but those on American fast food develop osteoporosis, even if they take a calcium supplement.

Let's take a look at the studies. Since recent media hype has led so many of us to overdo our calcium intake, this mineral deserves special mention.

- Dr. L. M. Resnick from Cornell found that high calcium levels in the body and low levels of magnesium contributed to high blood pressure, which causes a whole host of problems. Dr. M. Seelig reports that magnesium deficiency and at the same time a calcium overload causes coagulation within the arteries which makes the blood very difficult to pump and prevents it from flowing through the arteries. (Cows' milk is high in calcium and *low* in magnesium.) Higher levels of magnesium in the diet or lower levels of calcium can prevent these serious problems.

- Dr. W. B. Grant from National Aeronautics and Space Administration is concerned about male health, especially in situations of little exercise. He looked specifically at the impact of dairy products on coronary heart disease. In a study involving statistics from 32 countries, he found very high correlations between heart disease and the consumption of milk. For ischemic heart disease, he found the highest correlation with milk sugar for men over the age of 35 and women over the age of 65. Non-fat milk and coronary heart disease had the highest correlation with men over 45 and women over 75. Milk, sugar, and heart disease had the highest correlation for women between the ages of 45 and 64. He theorized that animal proteins contribute to homocysteine production but milk more than meat because it contains more methionine and lacks adequate B-vitamins to convert homocysteine into non-harmful products. Milk sugar and high calcium content may also contribute to calcification of the arteries.

• Drs. G. Fleckenstein-Grun and A. Fleckenstein from Germany found in doing human and rabbit studies that calcium plays a decisive role in human–type plaque formation. They found that calcium antagonists could partially overcome the problem of excessive calcium, but not all of them, without harmful side effects.

• To the rescue comes Dr. P. Raggi from Tulane University in New Orleans with a non-invasive testing method to find out if you have calcium deposits in your arteries that could block the flow of blood and cause death. The test is called "electron beam tomography" or EBT, for short. Several studies have shown that EBT is a very sensitive method to detect the calcification in the arteries that can lead to a high risk of death from heart disease. Dr. Raggi found that the density of calcium in the arteries was directly related to the severity of the plugging in the artery and of weaknesses in the wall of the artery. He also found the calcium density in the artery was directly proportional to the calcium and phosphate level in the serum, which of course comes from the diet-processed cheese, processed meats, phosphate loaded soda pop, and other processed foods. Many food companies add lots of phosphate to their products. Dr. Raggi found no correlation between calcification in the arteries and total cholesterol, HDL, LDL, or triglycerides. What Dr. Raggi has found was that some people have their arteries plugged with calcium and phosphate even though they have normal cholesterol values. Dr. Raggi predicts that tomography will become an important tool in predicting the effect of calcium and phosphate on soft tissues and the likelihood of having a heart attack, and in measuring the effectiveness of exercise, drugs or nutritional therapy.

• Drs. M. C. Kruger and D. F. Horrobin found that Omega-3 deficiency leads to development of severe osteoporosis and calcification in the arteries. Apparently, when the body is deficient in Omega-3, the body pulls calcium out of the bone and deposits it in the arteries. This arterial calcification is much more life threatening a disease than osteoporosis. They point out that Omega-3 increases calcium absorption from food, enhances the effects of vitamin D, reduces losses of calcium in the urine, increases calcium deposition in bone, and enhances the synthesis on bone collagen along with reduced deposition of calcium in soft tissues. Omega-3 helps you make the most effective use of the calcium.

Magnesium, Boron, Potassium and Sodium

The emphasis on calcium would make you think that it's all you need to make strong bones, but you would be very wrong to think so. Your diet must also contain adequate levels of magnesium and boron. The problem is that the standard American diet is extremely lacking in these minerals. You really need, at a minimum, to eat a lot of whole grains—but even then you might not be getting enough. Best of all is to eat whole grain foods that have been fortified with extra magnesium and boron. Most of all, you need to go back to Chapter 5 and consider upping your physical activity. *The real truth is that 80% of bone strength comes from weight bearing and bone-jarring exercise like doing pushups or lifting weights, brisk walking or jogging; not from the diet!* Remember that although exercise from swimming and biking is good for you, these activities will not strengthen your bones.

It's no wonder that so many people have bone problems since the modern American diet is so far out of balance and most people choose occupations that do not involve carrying extra weight around every day. This is the one advantage that obese people have over their skinnier friends and neighbors: they rarely have weak bones because they carry around a lot of extra pounds all the time, whether they want to or not. Becoming obese is *not* the best way to get stronger bones. You really need to get into regular activity like jogging, pushups, and lifting weights.

Magnesium is also extremely important for the healthy functioning of your heart. This is so thoroughly understood today that even a group of water bottlers have begun advocating for government-established minimum standards for magnesium in drinking water. Even so, most Americans simply don't understand the dangers of magnesium deficiency: according to the National Academy of Sciences, as many as 80% of us are deficient in magnesium and that correcting this deficiency could prevent up to 210,000 deaths from heart attacks a year. The FDA received this information in 1977 but has failed to take action.

There's lots of research on all of these important trace minerals and the role they play in maintaining heart health. Here are just a few that deal specifically with magnesium:

• Dr. Mildred Seelig, a dear friend of mine, has spent her whole life researching the role that minerals play in our health. In one of her studies, patient populations who were receiving long-term diuretic therapy also received magnesium supplements. The incidence of sudden cardiac death decreased for those receiving the magnesium. Lesions inside the arteries resulted from a lack of magnesium, a very early sign of heart trouble. Dr. Seelig found that if magnesium is low and calcium is too high, the blood can easily clot in the artery, causing a heart attack. Dr. Seelig found this could happen despite "normal" blood levels of calcium and magnesium, so one needs to do a magnesium-loading test to measure the total magnesium available in the body.

• Dr. G. A. Morrill and associates found that magnesium could prevent the burning of heart tissue by free radicals.

• Drs. A. Elamin and T. Tuvemo from Sudan found that due to the damage caused to the arteries as a result of magnesium deficiency, the incidence of diabetes increased. They recommended supplementing the diet of diabetics with magnesium.

• Dr. H. S. Rasmussen from Denmark suggests that all patients who have suffered a heart attack be given a supplement of magnesium directly into their veins because magnesium deficiency is so common amongst heart patients. He found that no drug on earth can make up for a nutrient deficiency and that there are absolutely no side effects from this treatment!

• Dr. C. D. Hix from New Jersey found that a decrease in magnesium is linked with irregular heartbeat, congestive heart failure, or heart attack conditions. He found that magnesium supplements are beneficial for treating and preventing life-threatening condition. These can be safely taken through the vein or through the stomach.

• Drs. C. A. Sueta and K. F. Adams Jr. from the North Carolina School of Medicine investigated congestive heart failure patients. Although therapy has progressed substantially, mortality heart failure is substantial, estimated at 60-80% per year. Due to magnesium's importance for the heart, he recommended that all heart patients should be monitored for magnesium and ones with irregular heartbeat should be given magnesium immediately.

Two other nutrients to keep in balance are sodium and potassium. In America, we consume way too much sodium and far too little potassium. As a result, we end up with congestive heart failure and a condition called edema, in which the body retains too much fluid in its tissues. If you've been troubled by the number of pounds showing whenever you step onto your bathroom scale, remember that many of the extra pounds may be caused by too much water in your tissues from consuming too much sodium!

The American diet is particularly heavy on sodium— and processed foods are usually very high in it even before you add your own from the saltshaker on the table. To get a good idea of just how much we tend to over-consume sodium, think about this: the body appears to need about 2,300 milligrams per day for optimal comfort and health, but Americans commonly consume between 9,000 to 15,000 milligrams! What's the price of this excess? Too much sodium can leach calcium from your bones, make you look and feel fat because of the bloating it promotes, and cause untold problems for your heart!

Why do food manufacturers go so heavy on the salt in their products? They love it because it's cheap, it's a natural appetite stimulant (making you crave more of their product), and can overpower unpleasant tastes from chemical additives or inferior ingredients. Additionally salt is a preservative, giving their products a longer shelf life. You don't need lots of salt to make your food taste good. There are healthy alternatives in the flavor-enhancing cupboard. Try replacing salt with fresh lemon pepper or other herbs and spices! If you commit yourself to a nutrition program based on fresh foods, you'll discover that they rarely need the kind of seasoning that processed foods demand.

If you simply can't cut out all the processed foods on the market today, you still have some options. Check the labels and buy only those that keep the added sodium down to the 100 to 150 milligram range. Above all don't load on more salt once you've put the food onto your plate!

Lets turn our attention to potassium and the role it plays in a healthy lifestyle. Once again, the evidence is impressive.

- Dr. J. G. Cleland and B. W. East studied patients with heart failure. They found that potassium deficiency was the main cause of irregular heartbeat and sudden death in Scotland.

- Dr. J. Constant of Buffalo New York State University found that magnesium couldn't work alone. In a study of patients with congestive heart failure, he found that some diuretics remove potassium, water-soluble vitamins and vitamin C from the body and that magnesium cannot work without these nutrients. This lowers the body's ability to deal with the stress of heart disease.

• Drs. D. H. Lawson and H. Jick reviewed a drug surveillance program that analyzed 3,879 patients admitted to the hospital with cardiac failure. They stated that potassium deficiency was very common in patients who were taking an aldosertone antagonist for their heart trouble.

• Drs. J. M. Potter and J. R. Cox demonstrated that potassium supplements could easily overcome potassium deficiencies in patients with heart failure.

• Drs. R. B. Singh and Z. Shoumin studied 3575 subjects ranging in age from 25 to 64 years, including men and women. They tracked their food intake and found a higher incidence of heart disease in people who consumed low amounts of zinc. These individuals also had higher blood pressure, higher cholesterol values, and a higher incidence of diabetes.

• Researchers from France found that as zinc levels went down, oxidative stress in the body increased. They found that zinc acted to increase anti-oxidant enzymes and prevented injury to the heart tissue if a heart attack occurred. Zinc also helped prevent second heart attacks.

• Danish researchers found babies born with heart problems usually had deficiencies of zinc, iron, calcium, and vitamins D, E, C, B-1, or B-6. They recommended that mothers-to-be take extra vitamins and minerals and to consume a healthy diet. They also recommended that parents give their children vitamin/mineral supplements.

• Drs. C. Coudray and A. Favier found that excess iron could cause production of excess free radicals and that zinc, copper, selenium inhibit the production of these free radicals. They found that excess alcohol could cause oxidation problems, and in the presence of zinc deficiency and iron excess, very serious problems could occur. In fact, it could cause the heart muscle to stop pumping.

• Drs. I. M. Hamilton and J. J. Strain found that copper deficiencies could lead to lesions in rat arteries and also lead to plugging of arteries.

• Dr. L. M. Klevay from the USDA Human Nutrition Research Center in Grand Forks found that excess iron could prevent copper from being absorbed and that copper deficiency can lead to heart attacks and osteoporosis. He recommends that an RDA for copper be established to prevent serious health problems.

Minerals and Heart Disease

In the case of heart disease, minerals like magnesium and potassium play vital roles. Without adequate levels of magnesium and potassium, especially when your diet contains too much sodium, your heart can drown by retaining too much water. If you're like many people who turn to the use of diuretics to reduce bloating, you just compound the problem. A long-term deficiency of magnesium and potassium can have truly dramatic consequences: it has been the cause of many cases of sudden, fatal cardiac arrest—especially among alcoholics and junk food junkies!

This is, in fact, what many people believe was behind the death of Jim Fixx, the famous long distance runner and author of *The Complete Book of Running*, which started the whole jogging craze in this country. Fixx was well known to be a big fan of junk food, and often bragged to the press that he could eat all he wanted because he could run off the extra calories. It's true that he stayed slim to the end of his days, but that was no protection for him. When he died he had such a bad case of hardened arteries that one of them was completely plugged up! Fixx's father shared a similar problem with cardiovascular disease, but go one generation further back and there's no evidence that the Fixx grandfather was troubled with such problems, so it can't be genetic. Instead, it's likely that Fixx learned some heart-unhealthy eating habits from his dad.

Unfortunately, Jim Fixx never seems to have looked beyond the calorie count when making food choices, and relied on his active athleticism to keep him lean. He probably never even knew that he was deficient in nutrients like magnesium and potassium. He learned the hard way that being a beloved author and/or an athlete does not guarantee clean arteries and good health.

Let's not make the same mistake that Jim Fixx did! Let's make the effort to look beyond superficial, "common knowledge" about nutrition and find out what we really need to stay healthy. That way we don't have to face the possibility of tragedy like the one that befell Fixx.

Recent research is beginning to turn up some pretty interesting information about potassium and strokes. Recently, scientists have found that insufficient levels of potassium may put people at a higher risk for strokes, especially if they are taking diuretics. If their theory is proven, some people may be able to reduce the danger of strokes by just changing their diets.

A study that appeared in the August 2002 issue of *Neurology* followed 5,600 men and women 65 and older from four to eight years. After keeping track of which people had strokes, Dr. Deborah M. Green and her colleagues of The Queen's Medical Center in Honolulu found that potassium appeared to have a role. They said people in the study with the least potassium in their diets were one and a half times as likely to have strokes as those with the most. A daily intake of 2.4 grams was defined as low, and 4 grams as high. Participants who were taking *diuretics* (medications that help fight high blood pressure, congestive heart failure, and kidney disease by flushing water out of the body) appeared to have a *higher risk*. The likely reason? While flushing excess water, diuretics also rid the body of potassium. Those taking the medication who had the lowest potassium levels were two and half times as likely to have strokes as those with the highest potassium levels.

Zinc, Iron and Copper

Other nutrients to keep in line are zinc, iron, and copper. Zinc helps keep your immune system healthy and your taste buds tasting, iron builds strong blood, and copper aids in the absorption of iron.

We all know that a deficiency of iron leads to a condition called anemia, but many people don't realize that an excess of iron can cause serious problems. Excess iron causes excess oxidation, resulting in the actual burning of your bodily tissues, leading to heart disease and cancer. In addition, it contributes to the formation of bigger, harder clots within the arteries, thus preventing the free flow of blood through your body!

Research on the problems of excess iron is well underway, with scientists reporting their findings from all over the globe. Here are some of the most important results found in the literature on the subject:

- Dr. K. Schumann from Germany found that *excess* iron causes compounds within the body to be oxidized, become toxic, cause cancer, and stimulate the growth of cancer cells. He also reported that excess iron increased the risk of diabetes and heart disease. His findings are corroborated by the research of Dr. G. F. Pool, reporting from South Africa. Pool has found that high levels of iron in men are also associated with an increase in LDL cholesterol.

• Dr. L. Y. Chau from Taiwan reported that iron is a main component of plaque deposits in the arteries. His study also showed that the more iron people consume, the more severe the arterial plugging.

• Dr. M. Roest from the Netherlands found that sometimes excess iron could affect multiple generations! His study of men and women whose fathers stored excess iron in their body as a result of a genetic defect, had over twice the normal rate of heart disease. In the men he studied, he also found very high rates of diabetes.

• Speaking of genetic conditions that cause the body to store excess iron: Dr. M. L. Rasmussen from the University of Minnesota did a study to investigate this problem. After adjusting for smoking, cholesterol level, diabetes, and other risk factors, he found that people with high serum ferritin levels had a 270 percent greater risk of having heart disease. This makes it important for those who have this genetic defect to give blood to reduce their stored blood iron levels.

• If you consume excess iron, you have to watch out for the "combination effect" of other food components. Dr. H. O. Mowri from Boston University found that excess sugar in the blood increased the damaging effect of excess iron to the arteries by four to six fold. Guess it is not a good idea to have that dessert after a big steak.

Here are some more important research findings about excess iron and its companion, oxidative stress:

• Dr. T. Inouo and associates at Dokkvo University School of Medicine in Saitama, Japan, found that the oxidation of LDL particles was twice as high in patients with heart disease than those without heart disease. The oxidized products caused a distinct progression of the disease.

• Dr. Paul Holvoet and colleagues from the Center for Molecular and Vascular Biology, Catholic University of Leuven, Belgium, found that measuring the oxidized LDL products would greatly improve the accuracy of predicting who would die from heart disease.

• Dr. Y. Yasunobu and associates from the First Department of Internal Medicine, Hiroshima University School of Medicine, Japan, found that oxidative stress was greatly increased in people with unstable angina – those on the verge of having a heart attack.

• Dr. S. Toshima and colleagues at Gunma University School of Medicine, Japan, found in their study of patients with heart disease that there was no correlation with total serum cholesterol levels and heart disease compared to the people who had no heart disease. They did find a direct correlation with heart disease and oxidized LDL particles.

• Dr. Fred Kummerow at The Burnsides Research Laboratory and The Harlan E. Moore Heart Research Foundation, University of Illinois, studied 1200 patients with plugged arteries and found that the extent of plugging did not correlate with the level of cholesterol in the blood. It did correlate with the level of oxidation products in the blood.

• Dr. P. Ebong at the Department of Biochemistry, University of Calabar, Nigeria, found that fresh palm oil containing high levels of saturated fats did not plug arteries, increase hardening of the arteries, increase blood pressure, or cause other health problems, but that oxidized palm oil caused many health problems. These included reproductive problems and problems in the heart, kidney, lungs, and liver. This is especially important in Nigeria because they use a lot of palm oil. They simply have to avoid cooking foods at high temperatures for long periods of time in rancid oil (deep frying).

• A study by Dr. H. van Jaarsveld from South Africa reports that stored iron (measured as serum ferritin) increased the level of LDL in the blood and increased the level of oxidized LDL, which greatly increases the plugging of arteries and the risk of having an instantly fatal heart attack. Another study found that excess dietary iron lowered the antioxidant level in the liver, red blood cells, and the blood stream, and also damaged the wall of the arteries. Excess iron also turned a small heart attack into a big one with a slow recovery.

• Dr. V. Herbert of the Nutrition Center in New York found that most free-radical injuries in the body start from excess iron floating in the system. He said this relates to increased risk of cancer and heart attack and other chronic degenerative diseases.

Like iron, zinc and copper are very important trace minerals since they are involved in hundreds of very important reactions in the body. They help all the other important nutrients do their jobs. They are involved in the sense of taste and smell, sexual potency, vision, the immune system, metabolism of Omega-3, and many other functions. Here too you need to avoid excess, especially because the two minerals need to be kept in careful balance. Too much zinc will produce a deficiency in copper just as too much copper will cause a deficiency in zinc. When you eat the fresh whole foods as grown from the earth, keeping these and other important minerals in balance is less of a challenge. Your second-best bet is to look for foods fortified with these minerals. Unfortunately, one of the best natural sources of zinc, along with pumpkin seeds, are oysters. I say unfortunately because, with the over harvesting of our oyster beds, I'd rather not find that my recommendation of these tasty morsels from the sea results in their overnight extinction!

Selenium and Chromium

Selenium and chromium are two more important trace minerals that you might not think about when planning your nutrition program. Selenium is important because it is a powerful antioxidant that helps prevent heart disease and cancer. Chromium is an important molecule because it helps the insulin molecule work efficiently to prevent diabetes. It acts to control the sugar metabolizing system so that we have enough energy at the right time, instead of being at the mercy of unexpected spikes and dips in our energy levels. In addition, chromium helps to keep the body burning sugar for energy instead of turning it into fat.

Making the Most of Your Minerals

Many people who are confused about the minerals they need in their diet, head for the supplement shelves at the local drug store, rather than try to fill their daily needs through natural sources. The best way to maintain the proper balance among all the minerals your system needs is to get them through the foods you eat. For magnesium, go for whole grains, seeds and nuts. For calcium, try fruits, nuts, seeds, vegetables and whole grains. Why go for synthetics when Mother Nature offers you what you need in such delicious forms? If you'd like a supplement, make sure it is a good, natural one.

What about sodium? It's unlikely that you're going to have a problem getting enough, but stay away from diuretics! Instead, avoid the highly processed (and therefore high sodium) foods and stick with fresh, wholesome ones. Then, instead of reaching for the saltshaker, try experimenting with other seasonings like red pepper and spices. Meanwhile, drink lots of pure water. Yes, that's right—drinking lots of water actually helps reduce the amount of water retained in your tissues because it *helps dilute and then flush away salt!* Remember, it's salt, not water, that actually causes puffiness and bloat.

CHAPTER ELEVEN

The WE-FOBAM Way

Back in the 1950s, when the Cholesterol Theory was first proposed, it caught on quickly with a medical establishment that was content to find simple answers to complex problems. It wasn't long before the MIC found ways to put the theory to profitable use, taking advantage of our very human desire to find short cuts to solve problems. We went along with it, even though their "solution" didn't reduce heart disease at all. Now we know better—and as the science makes ever clearer, even many members of the medical community are coming to recognize that cutting cholesterol alone will not significantly reduce the numbers of deaths and disabilities caused by diseases of the cardiovascular system.

Even as the science teaches us that heart disease has complex causes, calling for a more sophisticated, holistic solution, the profits continue to roll in for the MIC and its single-minded attack on cholesterol as the be-all and end-all of heart health. The MIC knows that as long as it can keep our fear of cholesterol at a fever-pitch, we'll keep lining up for their anti-cholesterol pills, and we'll keep filling the hospital rooms and operating theaters when we have our inevitable strokes, heart attacks, and other ailments. They have it made! They have no reason to find a better way, but you DO.

It's your health that's at stake here, and you now have the basic information you need to take control. In the previous chapters you learned of the many elements that contribute to good heart health, and they are all things that you can personally take charge of in your quest for a good, long, healthy life. "Knowing" is not the same as "knowing how." In this chapter, you'll learn how to take the knowledge of the WE-FOBAM program and put it into practice in your daily life. By so doing, you'll enhance the quality of your life and free yourself from the Cholesterol Terrorists once and for all.

Winning With WE-FOBAM

As you now know, the Cholesterol Terrorists have tried to convince us that all we need to do is pop a couple of anti-cholesterol pills a day and buy processed foods that say "Lite," "No Fat," or "No Cholesterol" and, like magic, we'll be healthy. You also know that this is a lie. What's more, in their single-minded efforts to terrify us about cholesterol, they've got us eating food that's either tasteless or so high in sugar and salt that we've nearly forgotten how good *real* food can taste. This is where you can make your first changes and join the WE-FOBAM way to a better life.

The Cholesterol Terrorists, and their tame Medical-Industrial Complex had their reasons for pushing their simplistic anti-cholesterol message, and those reasons really have nothing to do with a concern for your health. It's all about defending long-term profits and about making you dependent upon them—and their high-priced products—instead of taking charge of your own well-being. If you stick with their self-serving program, you lose—and you lose big!

You lose financially, because the way the cholesterol theory is set up, there's never any end to your reliance on their drugs, tests, and treatments. You lose in terms of your health, because your risk of coronary disease is unlikely to be reduced, no matter how many refills you get for your anti-cholesterol drugs. You lose personally, because you have relinquished control over your health. Finally, you lose in terms of the quality of your day-to-day life, because you deprive yourself of a wonderful new world of food and fitness that is yours for the taking!

With the WE-FOBAM way, on the other hand, all you can do is WIN! You become a winner financially because you are finally free of the need to throw good money down the bottomless pit of prescription drugs and medical services. You become a health winner because you make concrete, positive improvements in your physical condition, and dramatically reduce your risk of death or disability due to coronary disease. You win personally because you empower yourself, taking back the control over your health that should never have been taken away. When it comes to quality of life, you win your way through to a wonderful feeling of profound personal well-being.

Getting With the Program

The first thing you need to understand is that your body's needs are complex. There is no single "miracle" substance that will cure all your ills. That doesn't mean you have to rush out and acquire an advanced degree in biochemistry—it just means taking sensible measures to acquaint yourself with the important elements of a healthy lifestyle. This book is an important first step: you have begun to learn about the combination of nutrients required for a strong, healthy body, regardless of your age. With the knowledge contained in these pages, you can make healthy choices, even if you never take your research any further. On the other hand, you may find yourself energized by the sense of empowerment this basic knowledge gives you. If that's the case, you can use that inspiration to learn more, by visiting our website at www.realcauseofheartdisease.com, where we report on new science that may be useful to you in your quest for full, vibrant health.

The next step is to take what you've learned in these pages and put them into practice in your own life. Begin by taking stock of your usual diet and activity level. The tests at the end of Chapter 3 should help you there. Check out your own kitchen cupboards, refrigerator, and pantry. There are some things that should be a standard part of your daily fare for good, scientific reasons, that maybe you're neglecting. Remember, even if you recognize a need for exercise as a part of your new, healthier lifestyle, you are best off by starting with the nutritional element— you want to "tune-up" your vehicle (your body) before you take it out on the highway for a test drive! So let's recap what you can do to bring your body "up to speed."

Someone's in the Kitchen With WE-FOBAM

First, of course, you want to expand your food choices to maximize your WE-FOBAM intake. That is, you want to start making sure that you're getting plenty of water, Omega-3s, B-vitamins, fiber, antioxidants, and minerals. The best way to deal with the water is to retrain yourself to reach for it instead of high-sugar or caffeinated beverages. If you don't like the taste of water, that is no problem. Squeeze a little lemon or lime juice into your glass to add a slight tang. Get into the habit of carrying a bottle of water around with you, so you've got it handy.

Next you want to reconsider your dietary choices. What's wonderful is that many good, wholesome, fresh foods are great sources of more than one of the various WE-FOBAM nutrients. Whole grain breads, for example, are high in many of them, and if you choose bread that contains flax you've hit the Omega-3 jackpot as well. Colorful vegetables give you both vitamins and minerals, not to mention their high natural water content. Protein is necessary, of course, although not in the volume that Americans have become accustomed to, and you can get the animal protein you need without getting into a heavily meat-based diet if you allow yourself eggs and fish.

The beauty of the WE-FOBAM way is that it will probably introduce you to a whole new, more pleasurable, way of eating. If you've been living on the standard American diet of processed, packaged foods at home and fast foods outside, you're in for a treat: you won't believe how tasty whole, fresh foods taste!

Taking the WE-FOBAM Show on the Road

Making changes in something as basic as the way you eat can seem difficult, even overwhelming, at first. Remember all those studies we cited earlier? Many of them offer you great news for even a slow, gradual program of change. Increases in Omega-3s, for example, provide heart-health benefits even if you're still practicing other, less healthy behaviors, so does shifting from a lifetime practice of neglecting proper hydration to one that ensures that you get appropriate amounts of water every single day. In other words, you can phase in changes, allowing yourself the time you need to establish each new nutrient or practice as a regular habit before moving on to making the other necessary changes.

This is a good thing to know, because many of us have a hard time keeping up a new regimen of diet and exercise. We try to do it all at once, and if we're not ready for one part of it we're discouraged about the other parts. This is especially true when it comes to exercise. We start a new regimen of diet and physical activity, but our bodies haven't yet recovered from years of under nutrition and can't really handle the new levels of exercise. We end up feeling achy and tired, and decide it's too hard. So we quit the exercise, and soon we even find ourselves going back to the bad old ways of eating, too.

How much better our results would be if we took our time and made our changes gradually. We begin by making changes in our diet—and an easy, delicious way to do that is to incorporate whole-grains into every meal. Over time—and in a fairly short time at that—our bodies regain their proper balance of necessary FOBAM nutrients, and we're much more ready to step up our activity levels. In fact, you may even find yourself becoming more active without conscious planning. Your energy level will have raised enough to inspire your body to greater activity on its own!

A Note of Caution

Don't get me wrong. I'm not suggesting that you just take one element of the WE-FOBAM way. In the long run, you need it all. Even today, that's something the MIC and federal agencies (dedicated to your heart health) simply refuse to understand. Take the recent pronouncement by the American Heart Association on the subject of Omega-3s. The evidence that Omega-3 fatty acids are important for healthy hearts has finally reached such abundance that in late 2002 the AHA has finally had to acknowledge it, and the organization has released new recommendations suggesting that we should all be getting about 900 milligrams per day. Good news, right?

Well, it would be, except that this recommendation is as simplistic as the cholesterol theory was in the first place. It simply changes the nature of the "magic bullet" from anti-cholesterol drugs to fish-oil tablets. Remember the ultimate message of our WE-FOBAM approach to heart-health: you need all the nutrients: fiber, Omega-3s, B-vitamins, antioxidants, and trace minerals! Fish oil tablets take care of only one of these nutritional needs! Sounds suspiciously like another way to guarantee a market for a whole new pill industry, doesn't it?

Yes, Omega-3s are important. So are proper hydration, reasonable levels of daily activity, and all the other essential nutrients discussed in this book. Capsules will never be a satisfying replacement for whole, fresh foods. You want Omega-3s? Eat fish, if your lifestyle accommodates it. If you get tired of fish or if you're vegetarian, try whole-grain breads or drink mixes like Ultra Omega Balance that incorporate flaxseed—perhaps the richest plant-based source of Omega-3s available. In other words, keep your eyes on the big picture: your goal is to expand your lifestyle to incorporate fresh, whole-and-wholesome foods, daily activity to keep you feeling fit and strong, and water, water, water.

Nuts to Heart Disease

Perhaps the worst disservice that the Cholesterol Terrorists have done to us all is to make us afraid of whole categories of wonderful foods. It's probably not that they have anything against these individual food items—it's just that as long as they focus on cholesterol as the "evil-doer" for heart health, they have to condemn out of hand certain foods to stay consistent. One such maligned food category is summed up in a four-letter word: NUTS!

Nuts have been perceived for a long time as a high-fat, high-calorie food, to be avoided or to be consumed with strict moderation. That's Cholesterol Terrorist propaganda! The truth, borne out by research, is very different. According to the best scientific evidence, a daily helping of a handful of mixed raw nuts grown above ground is now considered an important part of a healthful, balanced diet,

The first reports celebrating the beneficial role of nuts came out in 1992, as part of the Adventist Health Study carried out by G. E. Fraser and collaborators at Loma Linda University in California, and published in the *Archives of Internal Medicine* in July of that year. Researchers noted that the dietary habits of Seventh-Day Adventists, a Christian group strongly represented in California, differ markedly from the American average.

They eat mostly cereal products, fresh fruits and vegetables, and little or no meat. Approximately 30 years ago, more than 30,000 Adventists agreed to participate in a multi-year study on their dietary habits and health status. They regularly filled out questionnaires, and the researchers thus had a long-term picture of how their food choices correlated with their physical health.

Over time, investigators noticed that nut consumption correlated with a lower risk of coronary heart disease. This finding came as a surprise, given the belief that the high-fat content of nuts had long been treated as a bad thing. The research was clear: individuals who ate nuts regularly had a 48 percent lower risk of fatal coronaries than individuals who ate nuts less than once a month. Men and women, vegetarians and meat eaters, older folk and younger ones alike experienced these fabulous results across the board.

Other epidemiological studies confirmed these results. The Iowa Women's Health Study, which was initiated in 1986, followed some 35,000 postmenopausal women who entered the study with no evidence of cardiovascular disease. Seven years of data later, the research showed that women who ate nuts two or more times a month were found to have a 19 percent reduction in the risk of CHD compared to those who never ate nuts. This was despite the fact that, in this population, the proportion of participants with high nut consumption was much smaller than in the Adventist Study.

The Harvard sponsored Nurses' Health Study, begun in 1980, corroborated these findings. This research followed more than 86,000 nurses for 14 years and found that those consuming five or more ounces (140 grams) of nuts per week had a 35 percent reduced risk for all forms of coronary heart disease, a 39 percent reduced risk for fatal coronary heart disease, and a 32 percent decreased risk for nonfatal heart infarction compared with those who consumed less than one ounce of nuts (28 grams) per week.

F.B. Hu and M. J. Stampfer of the Harvard School of Public Health reviewed the latest studies for the journal Current Atherosclerosis Reports in November of 1999 and confirmed these research findings. Their review also noted that the Harvard-sponsored Physicians' Health Study of 22,000 male physicians further supported the claim that nuts contribute to heart health. That study showed the risk of cardiac death decreased as nut consumption increased. Hu and Stampfer also highlighted the findings of the Cholesterol and Recurrent Events (CARE) Study, where the effect of nut consumption on recurrence of heart infarction was investigated. Participants who ate nuts at least twice a week had a 25 percent lower risk of recurrence of heart attack. Hu and Stampfer noted the remarkable consistency of the results of these five epidemiological studies, which covered very different populations. The beneficial effects persist when adjustments are made for other known risk factors, such as smoking, alcohol use, or lack of exercise.

Taking It to the Next Stage

The next logical question to ask is "Do all nuts provide this benefit, or are some nuts better than others?" This leads to a related question: "What is it in nuts that provides this apparent protection from heart disease?"

The only way to find out was to do more studies, this time trying to pinpoint the source of the benefits more closely.

This type of study is set up to compare the experiences of several groups of people, each of which is given a different regimen of nuts to consume, with one group given none at all (that is called the "control group"). The other groups are then differentiated by the kind of nuts they are given: some get mixed nuts, some get one of several specific kinds of nuts.

In one of the latest investigations of this kind by R. U. Almario and colleagues at the University of California-Davis, four groups of participants were created. Lets call them groups A through D. Group A consumed their normal diet (minus nuts). Group B got the same normal diet, with the addition of about 50 grams of walnuts per day. Group C got a low-fat diet, and Group D got a low-fat diet with a 50 gram walnut ration. In the July 2001 issue of the *American Journal of Clinical Nutrition*, the researchers reported their findings. Ultimately, they discovered that walnuts did indeed produce a beneficial effect on heart health. Other studies followed, testing different kinds of nuts. To date, about a dozen studies have evaluated the effects of "nut diets." These studies have varied in a number of ways:

- Almonds, walnuts, hazelnuts, pecans, pistachio nuts, and macadamia nuts have been tested

- The amount of nuts consumed per day varied

- Investigations have been carried out i̇
United States, some in Australia, New Zeȧ ⸺,
Japan, Turkey, and Spain

- Participants in some studies were healthy
adults, in some studies, they had heart health
issues

- In some studies, the basic diet was freely cho-
sen by the participants; in other studies, a
strictly controlled low-fat diet was prescribed.

What is astounding is that, regardless of the particular study protocol followed, every study came up with the
same general findings: a lowering of blood cholesterol
levels by about 5 to 15 percent as a result of nut consumption during a few weeks, with a similar effect on
LDL levels. HDL was unaffected in most studies. These
results compare very favorably with those achieved by
application of cholesterol-lowering drugs.

We still want to know just how nuts work their
magic. One possible explanation is that nuts are rich in
Omega-3 and monounsaturated fatty acids. Another is
that they have high levels of fiber, protein, and antioxidants. That means, in WE-FOBAM terms, that they provide 3 of the five major nutrient groups associated with
heart health. When it comes to choosing a snack food, this
means that nuts are a far better choice than the processed
munchies on the market. The only thing to keep in mind
is that, as in all things in life, you need to exercise moderation.

Hot Stuff

Here's another thing that the Cholesterol Terrorists ignore: there is an alternative to the high-sodium intake that characterizes many Americans' diets. They have convinced us to convert to processed "cholesterol free" foods and snacks, and ignored the fact that many of those so-called "healthy" options are often high in sodium. We all get far too much of that element in our diets, but there's a great way to cut it down without giving up on taste. Recent research has identified one long-overlooked flavor enhancer as an important source of a particularly heart-friendly nutrient. What is this special spice? Cayenne pepper!

Cayenne pepper—the stuff you put on your pizza or in ground form, use to season stews and sauces—contains a substance called capsaicin. A naturally occurring substance, it can't be patented by the MIC, so they can't jack up the price and make it profitable. That doesn't mean that it isn't worth including in your diet—it's amazingly good at unplugging arteries! You can buy it in capsule form at most herbal and health-food stores. You can also use it in your cooking? Its pungent flavor can add a whole new dimension to the taste of your foods, and it makes a great replacement for the salt. Don't just take my word for it. Listen to what the scientists have to say.

A Spicy Artery-Saver

Capsaicin's ability to improve the circulation system has been the subject of much recent research, which has found that the substance speeds up the delivery of oxygen and nutrients to every organ in your body. It has also gained something of a reputation for improving sexual potency. Not surprising, since users report that it enhances the function of every organ, from brain to muscles to lungs. The evidence available goes well beyond anecdotal reports of individual users.

A research team sponsored by Bristol-Myers-Squib suggests that capsaicin has helped to prevent irregular heartbeats and prevents arterial clogging. They also found that it worked without the side effects of conventional (that is, expensive, patented) drug therapies. In other words, it worked better than drugs that their own pharmaceutical teams were likely to come up with! Their findings were supported by research from China, which showed that the hearts of animals that suffered coronary events were protected from damage by capsaicin. According to this study, capsaicin worked by increasing the concentration of a compound in the blood (called CGRP) that is involved in the immune system's function. New Zealand researchers, intrigued by the CGRP blood compound, discovered that it is implicated in reducing the problems associated with heart failure, high blood pressure, cluster and migraine headaches, nerve damage, cold hands and feet, and many symptoms of menopause.

Other research disclosed additional benefits of capsaicin. It has been found to be a powerful agent for opening (dilating) the veins and arteries, to reduce insulin sensitivity and the circulatory problems associated with diabetes, and acts as a replacement for antihistamines. In addition it eases the problem of minor arterial hemorrhage after surgery. In short, it is becoming evident that capsaicin is one of nature's most profound healing substances—so you don't need to feel guilty about sprinkling it on top of your pasta salad. You don't even have to eat it to experience its beneficial effects—it works well even when it is sprinkled on a fresh wound, just after the bleeding stops (not before, because it does thin the blood somewhat, which delays clotting). It dramatically and visibly speeds up the healing process. I believe that Cayenne pepper capsules belong in every first-aid kit.

Are You Ready for a New Way

The WE-FOBAM way is your ticket to a new, more satisfying life. It offers you empowerment, it offers you control over your physical and personal destiny. And it frees you from the tyranny of the Cholesterol Terrorists and the MIC. With all these benefits, how can you go wrong?

CHAPTER TWELVE

Maximum Quality Of Life Plan

A maximum quality of life plan—what would that be for you? Most of us would include family, friends, satisfying work, financial prosperity, and a sense that our lives have meaning. I'm also sure that you will agree with me when I say that without your health, it is very difficult to truly enjoy the other blessings you have.

Adopting the WE-FOBAM approach can maximize your health. What's great about this is, like everything else in this world, it has a side effect. Unlike the side effects of the MIC-based approach to life, the WE-FOBAM side effect is entirely positive: while your health improves, so does your outlook on life, your effectiveness, and even your relationships! To realize these side effects, you have to remember to take it gradually. You want to incorporate long term, beneficial lifestyle changes that will stick with you over the long haul. To achieve this, you should introduce improvements on a slow, phased basis. Be like the tortoise – slow and steady wins the race.

Forget the Old Models

Nothing happens overnight. That's hard for most of us to accept in these days when immediate gratification is the goal, but we can't offer you that. Remember: you've taken a lifetime to accumulate the damage that you now hope to reverse. The good news is that this *can* be done—and it can be done relatively quickly. You won't wake up tomorrow with immediate visible results—but you will feel healthier and more vibrant within weeks!

With each gain in your health, you'll gain energy and a sense of increased well-being. This in turn will provide you with the inspiration you need to make further healthy changes in your life. It's like a self-sustaining motivational system: soon you'll find that your old way of doing things are less and less tempting. The desire to lapse back into bad habits will begin to disappear. The positive rewards of your new lifestyle will provide their own reinforcement, making this a lifestyle with which you can stick.

Believe and Be Healthy

Here's a truth that bears repeating: lifestyle changes are easiest to accomplish if you really believe they will yield rewards.   Nieca Goldberg, M.D. calls this the "Health Belief Model," first developed by psychologists who wanted to explain the factors that make people willing to adopt practices which were intended to improve their health. In her book, *Women Are Not Small Men, Lifesaving Strategies for Preventing and Healing Heart Disease in Women*, Doctor Goldberg identifies a set of attributes that contribute to the "health belief" that enables people to adopt changes in their lifestyle. These include:

- The perception that they are at risk for a certain disease

- They believe the disease can be serious

• They believe that the treatment or intervention will be effective

• They view the personal effort and cost of the intervention to be worthwhile.

Given the prevalence of heart disease in American society, nearly all of us perceive ourselves to be at risk—a fact that the MIC has taken shameful advantage of for decades. We all recognize just how serious cardiovascular disease can be, so it's the final two attributes that are important. This is the great thing about the WE-FOBAM way. If you educate yourself on the research about the nutrients your body needs, you can be certain that this "treatment or intervention"—good nutrition—will be effective. If you approach the program gradually, the effort and cost is more than worthwhile.

Health-belief isn't enough. Doctor Joseph Prochaska at Brown University has identified five key stages by which people make permanent lifestyle changes. These are:

1. Denial

2. Contemplation (considering making the change)

3. Preparation (making the commitment to change)

4. Action (taking steps to change)

5. Maintenance (making the change a part of your daily routine)

It is only after you've moved through all five stages that a change becomes a permanent part of your life. Obviously, the first stage is the hardest one to get through: denial that a change is required can keep you from even trying! But once you leave denial, you still have work to do. Contemplation and preparation are what this book is all about: in these pages you have been given "food for thought" that should help you recognize the need to make changes in your life, and you have also been given the information you need to make that commitment. Now is the time for action!

Remember stage five: maintenance. Old habits die hard, and it is easy to backslide. In fact, we're programmed for it. That fact is what the MIC relies on: it panders to our desire to find easy, no-effort solutions to our health issues by offering a miracle pill that promises to cure everything. That promise is false—and once you've made the commitment to a new, healthy lifestyle it will provide its own reinforcement.

The key is to make the changes gradually! Avoid going too long without food, and drink water often throughout the day. Going longer than 3 or 4 hours without food can allow a blood sugar drop, which causes your judgment to become impaired. You may grab something sweet, or caffeine, to 'boost' your energy—when in fact the opposite effect will occur. Stay hydrated and feed your body with small amounts of nutritious food often to keep your energy and spirits high.

An Example From the Diet Industry

The "get thin quick" fads out there provide a great example of how NOT to make a permanent lifestyle change. Check out the magazines in the rack when you are waiting in line for the cashier at your local supermarket. Just about every issue has a "lose 20 pounds in 20 days" diet featured on the cover. They may suggest starvation menus, lots of quirky fads, and (to keep their advertisers happy) lots of propaganda for the "low-fat" processed and packaged foods.

No one can stay on this kind of diet over the long term. Going on high protein, high fat diets can cause permanent kidney damage and severe bone loss. Cutting calories drastically–the way some of these diets recommend–just make you cranky, weak, and depressed. The only thing that *does* seem to stick is the reliance on processed foods—but that's because they're high in sugar, salt, and refined flour. The label "low-fat" means that the food itself has little fat—it doesn't tell you that your body will take the ingredients and *quickly turn them into fat in your body!!*

The fact is that the majority of Americans are carrying excess weight—almost all of us could stand to drop a few pounds. The solution is NOT to go on a fad diet. In fact, although the news is full of reports that obesity has become an epidemic over the last few decades, we've actually cut our average consumption of fats: from 40 percent of our calories in 1955 to 35 percent in 1995! Why are we so much fatter? Simple: we have become increasingly sedentary, and we eat foods that are quickly converted to fat. Take sugar. Sugar is entirely free of fat—but your body takes excess sugar and converts it into fat for storage! Refined, low fiber white flour products will also quickly convert into sugar in your body and it will be stored as fat in your body.

Where to Start

Your very first step, if you are taking prescription drugs for health conditions, should always be to talk with your physician. Tell him or her that you are making changes in the way you eat, but that you are NOT "going on a diet." Instead, tell your doctor that you are adding new foods, and that you believe that these may make a change for the better in your general health. Don't ask his permission to change your diet, but do ask him if healthy foods will interfere with the working of the drugs. If he says no, then you have the green light to go ahead.

Next, start incorporating some new foods into your daily diet. Notice that this is the opposite of what the "diet gurus" recommend. For them, the whole story is to avoid certain foods. In the WE-FOBAM program, we recommend the opposite: keep your regular foods for now, but just add a few whole, fresh foods as well, a little at a time. Once again, whole-grain breads and other baked goods are a good first choice for addition. The nutritional benefits are plentiful, and they have the added benefit of being immensely satisfying—dramatically cutting your cravings for the bad stuff!

After a few weeks, you'll probably notice a significant improvement in your general sense of well-being. You'll likely feel an increase in energy, and you may even begin to notice improvements in your mood and concentration. If you've been on medications up to now, talk to your physician about lowering the dosage of your prescriptions. For example, if you've been taking anti-cholesterol medications, you might ask to begin lowering them: your new dietary program will have probably significantly reduced the levels of cholesterol in your blood! If your physician gives you an argument about making such a change, consider consulting with a nutritionist as well: dietitians and nutritionists have studied the subject in far greater detail than most M.D.'s, and their recommendation might be helpful in getting your doctor to work with you.

A Day in the Life of Renewing Your Health

When you get up in the morning, don't go straight for the coffee maker. Instead, pour yourself a large glass of water. Next, have some fresh fruit, a couple of slices of bread, a bagel, or a bowl of whole-grain cereal. Sweeten the food with fresh fruit or a little real maple syrup. Only *after* that, if you still feel hungry, reach for the sweet roll. In other words, don't deny yourself that sweet roll in the very beginning—just postpone it until after you've had the good stuff!

At lunchtime, continue this policy of *additions*. No matter what you normally order, start out with a salad, soup, and some whole-grain bread. Once you've eaten them, feel free to order whatever you like—but ONLY if you still feel hungry. It is a good idea to include fish a couple of times a week for the Omega-3s.

Snacks are most people's downfall, whether salty or sweet. Don't forbid yourself the usual snack choices, but int of keeping nuts, fruits, veggie sticks, and ᴏᴛʜᴇʀ e foods at hand. You'll soon get into the habit of eating them simply because they're conveniently available!

For supper, keep it light. Remember—breakfast like a king, lunch like a prince and supper like a pauper. You won't sleep well or feel good with a stuffed stomach. Have a sandwich, bowl of soup, or some other light foods. Keep whole fresh fruit, freshly popped corn, or low-sugar granola handy for snacking if the urge occurs.

If you approach the change this way—by adding healthy options first, and only then turning to your old, familiar foods—you'll find it easy to increase nutritional intake without making yourself feel deprived. In no time at all you'll find that you have reached the goal: at least 5 nutritional whole grain products, perhaps some fish, fruits, five veggies and at least 6 glasses of pure water. The chart below shows you specific goals to aim for as you make your heart-healthy lifestyle changes:

W	Water	Six to ten 8-oz. glasses per day.
E	Exercise	30 to 60 minutes three times a week. Start slowly and increase gradually. Eventually include some fast workout, some weight lifting and lots of walking.
F	Fiber	Include 25 to 50 grams per day in your diet. Make whole grain foods the main part of your diet. Start gradually.
O	Omega-3	2,000 to 5,000 mg of Omega-3 daily. Use stabilized, fortified flax liberally in your diet and add fish if you are not a vegetarian.
B	B-vitamins	Get plenty of B-vitamins. Probably use a B-50 complex tablet.
A	Antioxidants	Get plenty of vitamin C from fruits and supplements. Get vitamin E from Whole grains and a supplement. Get lots of polyphenols from vegetables, whole grain and PAC sorghum.
M	Minerals	Eat plenty of fortified whole grain foods, whole fruit and vegetables.

If you're looking for a plan that will help you make the WE-FOBAM way a natural part of your life, we recommend one that was developed by the Oldways Preservation and Exchange Trust, which maintains an excellent website at www.oldwayspt.org. We've taken their recommendations and modified them to reflect our own experiences. Here are the principal points:

- Eating wisely can lead to vibrant, good health especially when you also maintain a healthy weight, exercise regularly, and drink plenty of water throughout the day.

- Eating for health is based on eating a large variety of whole foods. These foods are minimally processed whole grains, fruits, vegetables, legumes, nuts and seeds—regardless of culture.

- Scientific evidence is voluminous that people who have maintained traditional eating habits have a much better chance of maintaining good health than those who adopt fast foods and refined, processed factory-made convenience foods, which are fiber and nutrient poor.

- Fresh whole foods give you pleasure and enjoyment in your meals, whether you eat with friends and family or eat alone. You also understand that you are healthier and feel better when you eat whole foods most of the time, have feasting days just a few times a year and usually avoid fast foods altogether.

• Nutrition scientists praise traditional healthy patterns as the foundation for lifelong good health. These are the patterns established in all of the world's cultures by hundreds of generations of our ancestors. They represent some of the best food in the world, from Mediterranean to Asian to Latin American to Vegetarian. These are cultural models for healthy and delicious eating.

Getting Into Specifics

In practical terms, eating wisely means eating 1-3 slices of whole grain bread (preferably made with stabilized, fortified flax) at each meal, or a cup of rice or pasta, oats, corn, grain, sorghum. Tortillas, plantains, or skin-on potatoes (but not french fries) are also good. The key point is that these are whole foods. Refined foods, particularly refined grains like what you get in enriched white bread, are much more quickly digested, which can cause all sorts of problems, from overweight to constipation to stomach distress.

Eat More of Some Things

Eating wisely means making sure that you get a variety of whole fruits and vegetables throughout the day. The goal to aim for is about 5 cups per day. Aim for a mix: dark green, leafy vegetables as well as brightly colored ones. No single vegetable has all the nutrients you need, but a combination of colors, textures, and tastes vastly broadens the number and type of nutritional substances you'll be getting. While you're at it, go for a variety of fruits as well: apples, grapes, blueberries, cranberries, cherries, raisins, and plums—your taste buds will appreciate the range of tastes, and your body will appreciate the nutrients.

Get the majority of your protein in the form of whole grains, legumes, nuts, and seeds, as well as a little fish, chicken, eggs and soy products (including tofu and soymilk). Just keep the animal protein to no more than 3-ounces per day. These are all healthier choices than the red meat that so many Americans eat too much of these days. While we're on the subject of animal-based foods, here's another tip: moderate amounts of fat are necessary in your diet, but you should get most of it from plant oils and oilseeds (such as flax). Extra virgin olive oil, for example, is better than any other kind of oil. Hydrogenated fats are the absolute worst choice you can make. Eventually, you want to get to the point where you can skip deep-fried foods entirely, for these are heavily laden with trans-fats and hydrogenated fats. Avoid bread products that contain partially hydrogenated fat, as they are harmful trans fats!

Eat Less of Other Things

Another long-term goal is to reduce your sugar and salt intake. They provide you with little or no physical benefit, and in fact can cause serious health problems. Once you become acquainted with the great taste of whole, healthy foods, you'll wonder why you used so much sugar and salt in the past! Don't forget that if you need to "spice up" a dish, pepper (particularly cayenne) is a great choice. Replace soft drinks with natural fruit juices or water. While alcohol in excess is never a good idea, moderation (the equivalent of no more than one drink per day) can actually provide some health benefits. Just remember that in hot weather alcohol can be a dangerous choice because it causes dehydration.

Finally, you should be aiming to minimize your consumption of dairy products. This flies in the face of "conventional wisdom" because we've all been taught that you need milk for strong bones and teeth. In fact, your body does need calcium, but there are far better sources than mucous-forming, high protein cows' milk and products made from it. You're much better off turning to green leafy vegetables and fortified whole-grain breads for the calcium in your diet, and strengthening your bones with weight-bearing exercises.

One extra benefit of this whole "eating wisely" approach (in the next chapter) is that you will find yourself getting more directly involved in the preparation of your meals. For many people, this is a wonderful new experience–part of the celebration of life. You will come to discover greater pleasure in your meals, whether you share the experience with friends and family, or dine quietly on your own.

A More Direct Approach

My own involvement in nutrition has been a lifelong affair. How lucky I have been, however, to have the support and partnership of my wife, Barbara Reed Stitt, in this endeavor. Like me, she has made the advancement of healthy nutrition a central part of her life. In her book *Food and Behavior*, she offers several useful tips for those having emotional or behavior problems in school and wanting to improve learning ability. It's the best book I have ever read and, of course, I am not prejudiced.

Barbara's approach (in the next chapter) is based on twin goals—feeling better and behaving better. On one hand, she recommends making certain additions, such as water, exercise, and particular food groups rich in nutrients and fiber. On the other hand, you want to remove from your body harmful substances that lead to poor health. Each goal is important in its own right. The long-term goal is the same, whether you take her direct approach or the more indirect, gradual approach discussed earlier: to maximize the quality of your life through wise nutrition and improved fitness.

– CHAPTER THIRTEEN –

The Actual WE-FOBAM Eating Plan

Eating wisely can lead to vibrant, good health especially when you also maintain a healthy weight, exercise regularly, and drink plenty of water throughout the day.

Eating for health is based on eating a large variety of whole foods. These foods are minimally processed whole grains, fruits, vegetables, legumes, nuts and seeds—regardless of culture.

Scientific evidence is voluminous that people who have maintained traditional eating habits have a much better chance of maintaining good health than those who adopt fast foods and refined, processed factory-made convenience foods, which are fiber and nutrient poor.

Fresh whole foods give you pleasure and enjoyment in your meals, whether you eat with friends and family or eat alone. You also understand that you are healthier and feel better when you eat whole foods most of the time, have feasting days just a few times a year and usually avoid fast foods altogether.

Nutrition scientists praise traditional healthy patterns as the foundation for lifelong good health. These are the patterns established in all of the world's cultures by hundreds of generations of our ancestors. They represent some of the best food in the world, from

Mediterranean to Asian to Latin American to Vegetarian. These are cultural models for healthy and delicious eating.

Wise Eating Dietary Advice For Individuals and Families

1. **To eat wisely means to eat whole grain foods and related foods that are minimally processed.**

    a. A good amount of grain is 1 to 3 slices of whole grain bread, made with flax, at each meal or   a cup of rice or pasta, oats, corn, grain sorghum, tortillas, plantains, potatoes (not french fries) or other cereals.

    b. Whole grains are digested gradually to prevent blood sugar fluctuations.

    c. Highly refined grains (i.e. enriched white bread) are digested rapidly, which can cause overeating, stomach problems, weight gain, and constipation.

    d. Cooked breakfast cereals can be a healthy start for the day, if they are minimally processed and not loaded with sugar or fat.

2. **Eat a variety of whole fruits and vegetables throughout the day.**

    a. Variety means different kinds of fruits and vegetables of all shapes, colors, textures and tastes.

b. An excellent amount of fruits and vegetables is about 5 cups per day.

c. The greatest health benefits come from eating lots of cooked and raw fruits and vegetables each day. Salads are best when made with dark greens mixed with vibrantly colored vegetables such as radishes, red and orange peppers, etc.

d. Frozen fruits and vegetables are good to eat when fresh are not available, especially if sugar, salt and fat have not been added.

e. Fruits and veggies are great snacks. These include apples, grapes, celery and carrot sticks, and dried fruits such as apricots, plums and raisins.

f. When possible, eat local, seasonal and fresh fruits and vegetables.

3. **Wise eaters eat protein mostly as whole grains, legumes, nuts and seeds, fish and chicken.**

a. Eating enough whole grains to obtain 25 to 40 grams of fiber will provide about half of your requirement for protein.

b. Legumes are beans, lentils, peas, peanuts and soybeans. Dried beans, peas, and lentils are regular sources of protein throughout the world. Nuts and seeds are protein-rich and delicious, healthy, convenient snacks.

c. Enjoy eggs, soy, tofu, and soymilk or rice milk once or twice a day in place of meat.

4. **Eat moderate amounts of fat, preferring plant oils, and oilseeds such as flax, over animal fats.**

   a. Extra virgin olive oil is preferred over other oils.

   b. Enjoy baked foods made with flaxseed, for its Omega-3 content, or sunflower oil or canola oil.

   c. Always AVOID foods made with partially hydrogenated fats.

   d. For cooking, use virgin olive or sesame oils instead of corn oil, safflower oil, butter, lard, beef or pork fat.

   e. For salad dressing, use olive, peanut, sesame or canola oils and other seed oils.

   f. Always AVOID deep-fried foods as they are heavily laden with trans fats and hydrogenated fats.

5. **Keep the amounts of added sugar and salt to a minimum.**

   a. Avoid soft drinks, fruit drinks, colas, candies, ice cream, fast foods and other related foods that are laced with artificial sweeteners, colors or sugars.

b. Use salt sparingly and avoid salt-laden snack foods, fast foods and processed meats.

c. Prefer raw or lightly salted nuts, fresh and dried fruits as your snack foods.

d. Allow yourself to understand the difference between natural fresh or frozen fruit juices and fruit drinks made with sugar and artificial coloring.

6. **Wise eaters drink 6 to 10 glasses of water a day and drink alcohol in moderation.**

a. Moderation is no more than one alcoholic drink a day.

b. Responsible drinking takes place at a meal or in social settings with friends and family.

c. Drink water throughout the day, especially in hot weather because you understand healthy bodies need lots of water and that you should drink water even if you do not feel thirsty.

7. **Enjoy the pleasures of your food and meals.**

a. Prepare your own foods often and you'll find that your 'hands on' contact with your food is part of the celebration of life.

b. Enjoy eating with friends and family at meals, and at other times enjoy a quiet meal by yourselves.

c. Boil, broil, bake, roast, steam, sauté or stir-fry your foods to reduce added cooking fat.

d. Take time to shop and read labels because you want to know what your foods contain and where they come from.

e. Wise shoppers let their friends know when they find especially fresh, nutritious foods.

8. **Wise eaters are concerned about their bones and joints.**

a. You should know that there is no convincing evidence that dairy users have fewer bone fractures than those who avoid dairy products.

b. Most modern dairy farms make cows suffer with shortened lives and poor health from being injected with bovine growth hormones, antibiotics and other drugs, which are passed on to humans. (Have you noticed the early maturation of children and how much taller each generation has become?)

c. Most factory farms have cows standing in manure all day. The milk may be contaminated with manure and is likely to contain harmful bacteria and virus.

d. Cheese, with no fiber, tastes good but it can make you overeat — especially overeat protein.

e. Wise eaters know that little calcium is retained if the diet is high in salt, fat, and protein, and that milk exacerbates diabetic symptoms.

f. Weight bearing exercise like pushups and pull-ups or weights is what strengthens bones.

g. For good health, know that calcium from leafy green vegetables and from breads fortified with calcium, are excellent, non-mucous forms your body can use without developing calcification in your joints and arteries.

h. Ask yourself, "What does a cow eat to get calcium? Does she drink milk and eat cheese, or does she eat vegetation? Once a baby elephant is weaned, what does it eat to grow all those huge bones — with no arthritis or osteoporosis? It eats leaves and grass." No other species drinks milk after it is weaned, and no animal drinks milk from another species – only people – because it is a huge business. Eat your dark green leafy vegetables and whole grains!

Vibrant Health

The following is a more direct approach to teaching one how to eat better to have Vibrant Health. My wife, Barbara Stitt, author of *Food & Behavior*, developed this plan.

Add to Your Body:

- **Water** – Drink 6 to 10 glasses of pure water daily. **Why?** Helps keep your blood flowing, your brain cells floating in 85% water, flushes out toxins, helps keep all organs and joints lubricated.

- **Exercise** – at least 1/2 to 1 hour daily. **Why?** Helps keep your body flexible and youthful, helps stabilize your weight, and have good circulation for sustained energy. Enjoy stretching, walking, jogging, yoga, biking and use weight bearing exercises to keep your bones strong and your muscles toned. *(A simple formula that works: walk as fast as you can as far as you can.)*

- **Fruits** – all kinds and all colors – fresh or frozen. **Why?** These most natural of foods for your body helps keep you in alkaline/acid balance, potassium balance, provides cleansing fiber, vitamins and minerals...delicious and beautiful. Wonderful in smoothies, too!

- **Vegetables** – fresh or frozen and especially eat dark green leafy and colorful vegetables. **Why?** Helps keep your eyesight sharp and sparkling, high in good fiber, high in vitamins and minerals, including the magnesium and calcium your body can use for strong bones. Enjoy fresh vegetable juices!

• **Whole Grains** – Wheat, oats, flax, brown rice, high lysine corn, etc. **Why?** Excellent sources of fiber, vital B-vitamins (found in the bran and germ), protein and minerals. The satisfying fiber in plant protein helps to *keep your daily intake of protein between 45 – 50 grams* for better calcium balance from the vegetables. Flax is the best possible source of Omega-3. You need 3 – 5 grams per day if you have heart disease or cancer.

• **Nuts & Seeds** – Flaxseed, walnuts, pecans, almonds, sunflower seeds, pumpkinseeds, etc. **Why?** Excellent sources of essential fatty acids, omega-3, vegetable protein, fiber, vitamins and minerals that keep your heart healthy and helps control blood sugar. Fresh nuts and seeds mixed with a little dried fruit makes a satisfying snack.

• **Legumes** – beans, peas, lentils. **Why?** They provide your body with essential nutrients, good plant protein, and high fiber that helps prevent the buildup of toxins and heavy metals (such as lead). Legumes give long-term energy and satisfy your hunger.

• **Good Fat** – Extra Virgin Olive Oil, Flax Oil, Canola Oil, Sunflower Oil, Avocado and cold water fish such as tuna, salmon and sardines. **Why?** Your body needs good fat that provides essential fatty acids such as Omega-3 to keep you skin, hair, and eyes glowing. Good fats also help keep your joints and organs operating smoothly...about 15% - 20% of your daily calories. Did you know that 60% of brain tissue is composed of essential fatty acids and your brain suffers if you don't consume it?

NOTE: *If you have Blood Sugar problems (high or low) – eat small amounts of the above foods 5 to 6 times daily. Your body can properly digest smaller amounts of food and be able to use all of it for energy. When your blood sugar drops you will have a tendency to overeat and/or crave sweets. If you are allergic to any of the above foods – simply avoid that food.*

Remove From Your Body:

• **Sugar** - the first addiction! Starts out as a food but it is refined down to just the sweetness – with no fiber or nutrients to slow its entering your blood stream. When your pancreas tries to limit the amount of sugar getting to the brain, it thinks the sugar will continue coming into your body at the same rate so too much is turned into glycogen and stored as fat – leaving your body in the state of "low blood sugar." Low blood sugar can trigger anxiety, irritability, sluggishness, headaches, depression, etc. and can lead to diabetes –turning your life upside down and miserable...so don't do it to yourself!

• **Artificial Sweeteners – Increase your desire for sweets and bad fats by 300%!** If you doubt this, go off your "diet soda" for a week or so and then have some and find out how hungry you get. Artificial sweeteners have been found inside brain tumors...which just could be the result of your body trying to get it out of your blood stream.

• **Caffeinated Beverages** – gradually cut down as they have a dehydrating effect and large amounts can cause jitters, irritability, insomnia and elevated blood pressure. If you want something hot, try hot water with fresh lemon – it's delicious. Scientific studies have found that *even five glasses of water daily can cut the chance of heart disease by 50%.* However, it has also been shown that just **five - eight ounce servings of other drinks can increase your chance of heart disease by 257%.**

• **Partially Hydrogenated Fat** – high in *trans* fats, which scientific studies show is a high contributor to heart disease, cancer and obesity. Trans fats are in all fast foods. Read labels!

• **Foods Made With Refined, Enriched White Flour** – almost no fiber allowing it to quickly turn into glucose in the blood stream. When coupled with sugar, lactose sugar, and/or caffeine, your body will quickly undergo severe stress due to the loss of B-vitamins and other nutrients, contributing to low blood sugar.

• **De-emphasize Animal Products** – Consume no more than 3 ounces two or three times weekly for best health.

• **Cigarettes** – Cause even higher rates of cancer and heart disease than formerly thought. For natural help to cease smoking in seven days call 1-800-704-1210.

• **Alcohol** – Can cause rapid fluctuations in your blood sugar and mood swings. In excess, can lead to addiction, emotional problems, gastritis, ulcers, pancreatitis, hepatitis, cirrhosis of the liver, hypoglycemia, diabetes, gout, and nerve and brain dysfunction. A little wine occasionally may be good for your health ...but red and purple grape juice does about the same thing.

Remember: *When you realize you should change your diet for better health, do it gently, lovingly and gradually. Even one soda or cup of coffee per day can cause headaches if stopped abruptly – so cut it down by four ounces each four days until you are down to zero per day.*

Our Personal Quest

No matter what approach you take in your quest for better health, one of the easiest ways to dramatically improve the nutritional content of your diet is to add fortified *whole-grain* baked goods: they're tasty, most of them require little or no additional preparation, and they offer a wide range of the nutrients your body needs, including fiber and Omega-3s, vitamins, minerals and antioxidants. If you are allergic to grains, move to other plant foods to replace the grains like brown rice, etc. Not so long ago, there were very few sources of these well-balanced baked goods, but in recent years specialty bakeries have begun springing up all around the country. We want to help promote all true, whole grain bakeries and would encourage all of them to incorporate stabilized, fortified flax in their products. Natural Ovens' sister company, ENRECO Inc., can help. Their web site is www.enreco.com.

My wife and I were early pioneers in the fortified whole grain movement. I founded Natural Ovens Bakery in 1976 and Barbara joined me in 1982, when we were married. At first we were a local phenomenon, but eventually we expanded to shipping whole grain foods throughout the Midwest and beyond. Someday, our products may be available at a store near you. Today we ship our products, books and videos nationwide through telephone orders (call 1-800-772-0730) or through our website (www.naturalovens.com). The website also offers nutritional information and an excellent cookbook that will help you expand your healthy choices in nutrition.

The Final Word

Together, Barbara and I have devoted our careers to spreading the word about healthy nutrition, and to helping people like you to take control of their lives. We've even extended that goal to our business. When we die, we have arranged a trust that will turn our Natural Ovens Bakery over to the control of our employees so that the mission can continue on even after we have gone. What started out as a strictly local enterprise has grown, in part, because most people really are hungry—not just for food but for empowerment. We want nothing more than to help you learn what you need to know in order to help yourselves. As you grow in the WE-FOBAM program, we welcome you to participate more fully in our goal. You can do this by visiting our newest website, www.realcauseof-heartdisease.com. There you'll find the latest scientific research on nutrition. Working together, we can all learn to maximize the quality of our lives, and spread the word to others as well.

We wish you vibrant health and would enjoy hearing about your own success. You can email us at info@realcauseofheartdisease.com

My wife and I wish you the very best!

**May all the rest of your years
be the very best years of your life!**

Heart Health Food "Starter Kit"

To be sure you get started with foods high in fiber, Omega-3, vitamins, minerals, antioxidants, and good taste, we have put together this "Starter Kit." Please call 1-800-772-0730 to order and you will be able to talk to a real, live person.

1 loaf Hunger Filler Bread............................$3.20

1 loaf Health Max Bread.............................$3.20

1 pound Ultra Omega Balance $9.75

1 package Gourmet Dinner Rolls................$2.50

1 package Brainy Bagels.............................$2.60

1 package Chocolate Raspberry Cookies $3.20

The Natural Ovens Cookbook....................$12.00

Subtotal............................$36.45

Ground Shipping..............$10.50

Total.................................$46.95

Special **Just For You!**........**$39.00**

For other Natural Ovens Bakery products, please check out our website at:
www.naturalovens.com

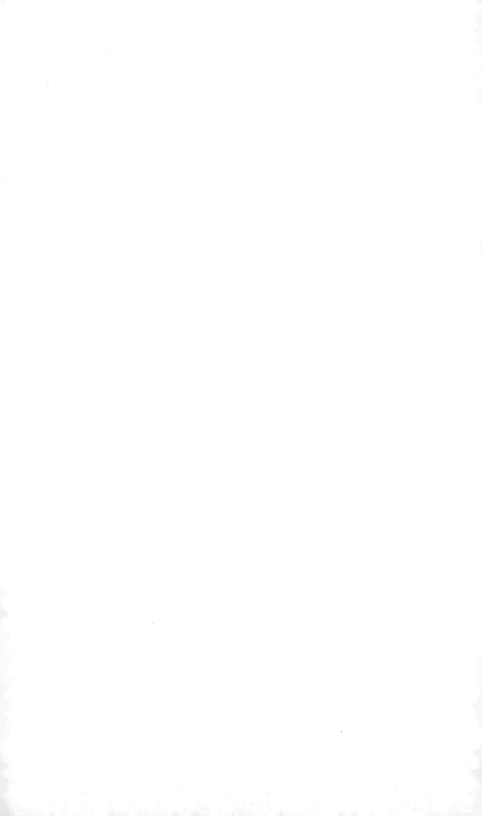

Recommended Reading

Stitt, Paul A. *Beating the Food Giants*

Stitt, Paul A. *Why George Should Eat Broccoli*

Stitt, Barbara Reed *Food & Behavior*

Stitt, Barbara *The Natural Ovens Cookbook*

Burke, Jeanie, R.D.
Vegetarian Cooking With Jeanie Burke, R.D.

Diamond, John, M.D.
Facets of a Diamond: Reflections of a Healer

Dufty, William *Sugar Blues*

Felix, Clara
The Felix Letter: A Commentary on Nutrition

Joseph, James A., Nadeau, Daniel A. and Underwood, Anne
*The Color Code: A Revolutionary Eating Plan for Optimum
Health*

Malkmus, George H., Dr. *God's Way to Ultimate Health*

McDougall, John A., M.D.
The McDougall Program: Twelve Days to Dynamic Health

Minsky, Bonnie C. *Our Children's Health*

Rudin, Donald, M.D. and Felix, Clara
Omega-3 Oils: A Practical Guide

Schlosser, Eric *Fast Food Nation: The Dark Side of the
All-American Meal*

Schmidt, Michael A. *Brain-Building Nutrition: The Power of
Fats & Oils*

Simopoulos, Artemis and Robinson, Jo *The Omega Plan*

Index

A

Alcohol
  Detrimental to your body, 201
  Maintain moderation, 187–188

American Heart Association
  Support of cholesterol theory, 2
  Inclusion of Omega-3 in
  dietary requirements, 50

Anti-cholesterol drugs
  Downside, 45–46

Antioxidants
  Benefits for the body, 127–128
  Beta-Carotene, 127
  Catechins, 128
  Flavonoids, 128
  Isoflavones, 128
  Polyphenols and heart disease, 128
  Proanthocyanidins, 128
  Science, 129–135
  Sources of Beta-carotene, 137
  Sources of phyoestrogens, 137
  Sources of polyphenols, 137
  Sources of vitamin C, 137
  Sources of vitamin E, 137

Arrhythmia
  Caused by Omega-3 deficiencies
  in the heart, 100

Artificial sweeteners
  Increase desires for sweets and fats, 199

D

E

F

L

M

O

P

Polyphenols
. *see* Antioxidants

Potassium
. *see* Minerals

Proanthocyanidins
. see Antioxidants

Pyridoxine
. *see* B vitamins

R

Refined, enriched white flour
Impact on the body, 200

Responsibility for health
Potential of the individual, 40

Responsibility for health
B vitamins, 126
Winning with WE-FOBAM, 163

Riboflavin
. *see* B vitamins

S

Selenium
. *see* Minerals

Sodium
. *see* Minerals